Minding My Mitochondria

How I overcame secondary progressive multiple sclerosis (MS) and got out of my wheelchair.

Terry L. Wahls, M.D.

Includes Over 100 Recipes for a Healthy Brain!

A practical guide to understanding mitochondrial health and the steps you can take to improve your brain's function and health.

2nd Edition

TZ Press, L.L.C.
Iowa City, Iowa

Illustrator: Tom Nelson. Cover illustration by Gary Carlson; gifted by Darlene McCord, Ph.D., FAPWCA, Pinnaclife, Inc.

Published by: TZ Press, L.L.C., Suite #101
1215 Santa Fe Drive, Iowa City, Iowa 52246-8637, U.S.A.
Single copies may be ordered from TZ Press L.L.C. Quantity discounts are also available. Please indicate the quantity of books you wish to purchase. Special books or excerpts can be created to fit specific needs. For details, contact TZ Press, L.L.C.

The body text for *Minding My Mitochondria* is set in APHont™, a font developed by the American Printing House for the blind, specifically for low-vision readers. APHont embodies characteristics that have been shown to enhance reading speed, comprehension, and comfort. For more information, visit www.aph.org.

Special thanks to the Vitamix corporation for permission to reproduce and reprint several beverage recipes, as designated in the text. The Food Function Chart, Sample Menus, and Daily Logs are all reprinted with permission from the Wahls Way © 2009 and may be reproduced for personal use only.

Printed in the United States of America
ISBN 13: 978-0-9821750-8-8
ISBN 10: 0-9821750-8-6

Foreword

No specific cause/etiology for multiple sclerosis has yet been identified. However, contributing factors such as environment, viral, immune dysregulation, and genetic predisposition have been linked to the disease. MS is considered to be an autoimmune disease in which the body's own immune system attacks the central nervous system.

Dr. Wahls was initially diagnosed with multiple sclerosis, relapsing-remitting type, in 2000 at The Cleveland Clinic. She was treated with different disease-modifying medications for MS. By 2003, her MS had transitioned to secondary progressive MS with relapse. She had multiple problems, including difficulties with walking, poor balance, and poor coordination. She had to use a cane or ski pole to assist with ambulation and a scooter and then a tilt-recline wheelchair for longer distances. Over the next three years, she gradually became weaker.

Dr. Wahls researched the nutrient requirements for the brain and mitochondria and began creating an intensive nutrition program for herself. Then she learned about a research study using neuromuscular electrical stimulation in people paralyzed by traumatic spinal cord injuries. In 2007, she revamped her diet to ensure that every calorie would contribute to maximizing the brain's building blocks and convinced her physical therapist to begin treating her with neuromuscular electrical stimulation. In less than a year, she was walking without a cane and could even bicycle. Her dramatic recovery without the use of drugs is impressive.

We know about the positive effects of good nutrition on many disease processes, including MS, and the benefits of physical therapy, exercise, and neuromuscular electrical stimulation in maintaining and restoring strength. Dr. Wahls was the first to combine all these measures. Likely, it was the synergy of all of her interventions that led to her stunning recovery.

The past 20 years have seen major changes in the ways MS is diagnosed and treated. Although a reduction of exacerbations may result from the new drugs, their ability to arrest the progression of the disease remains in question. Dr. Wahls has provided us with a book that covers the whole range of issues involved in this complex disorder. Too many physicians do not understand the critical role nutrition plays in brain health. This book is a valuable resource for physicians, MS patients, and their families to learn how to eat for optimal brain health. Eat well and mind your mitochondria.

E. Torage Shivapour, MD
Professor of Neurology, University of Iowa Carver College of Medicine

CONTENTS

Chapter One
THE BEGINNING

The rising costs of health care are crushing us. The magnitude of this increase is the result of more than just our aging populace, and therefore, an increase of diseases associated with old age, such as diabetes, heart disease, arthritis, and cancer. Over a third of our children either are or are projected to become burdened with serious medical conditions like autism, depression, learning disabilities, obesity, or pre-diabetes, many of which require expensive, lengthly treatments and programs.[1-15] However, despite all the money we spend on health care—more than any other country in the world—we are, as a nation, progressively less well.

Why is this happening to us? What has given rise to the single largest epidemic of chronic disease in human history? Have our genes gone bad? After all, scientists are identifying more genes associated with chronic disease each day. Are genetic mutations transforming our strong, lean bodies into obese, chronically diseased ones, or is there something else going on that is causing this change in the health of our country?

I think the explanation for what has been happening can be found in the cornfields of Iowa. When farmers buy seed corn, all the kernels in the bag of seed corn will have essentially the same DNA, the same genetic code, so the farmers know what kind of crop to expect in the fall. Say a farmer plants half of the bag of seed corn in rich, black Iowa soil and the other half in a trash heap filled with plastic debris and rock. When the farmer returns in the fall to harvest the corn, the corn planted in the black dirt will be tall with three ears of corn on every plant. But the corn in the trash heap will look diseased. Instead of being dark green, the corn stalks will be yellowed and stunted. Few stalks will have an ear of corn and only a few kernels will be present on each. It was the same seed, with the same DNA, in both locations. But the black Iowa dirt was filled with the nutrients needed for the corn's optimal growth. A trash heap lacks nutrients, and as a result, the corn grew poorly. It's through this simple example that we can answer the most pressing medical question of our time.

All living things, including our bodies, break down with time. Fortunately our bodies have tiny little maintenance workers inside our cells called mitochondria, which are busy supporting our cells doing the repair of the wear-and-tear damage that naturally occurs each day. Our DNA provides the blueprint for all the proteins and other biological components that need to be replaced on a regular basis. If those little maintenance workers don't have all the proper nutrients, like amino acids, the correct minerals, and fatty acids, then they can't build according to the DNA blueprints. Those nutrients are the building blocks that mitochondria in our cells need to keep our bodies healthy. If those replacement molecules and structures get made incorrectly or not at all, our bodies begin to deteriorate.

Instead of eating healthy food filled with micronutrients, most of the children in the United States regularly drink sugared beverages and rarely eat even one cup of vegetables or fruit with a meal. Micronutrients are the minerals, vitamins, and other substances that are essential, even in tiny quantities, for our growth and metabolism. Most adults do no better. The building blocks needed by our cells to maintain our bodies—micronutrients—are virtually absent from the standard American diet. As a result, our bodies become weaker at the cellular level, we lose our vitality, and we become far more susceptible to chronic diseases like obesity, heart disease, and even Alzheimer's.

Concerns about dietary cholesterol and sodium are frequently discussed on TV and the Internet, but of more important concern for most of us should be the amount of micronutrient content in our food. Leafy greens and non-starchy vegetables, fruit, fish, and meat from grass-fed animals supply the building blocks our cells desperately need.

Previous generations easily ate nine cups of vegetables and fruit each day. So should we. Three cups should be green leafy vegetables like spinach, romaine lettuce, or collards. Three cups should be brightly colored vegatables such as beets, red cabbage or carrots, or fruits like berries, oranges, or watermelons. Eat three more cups of your choice of vegetables before eating any kind of starchy vegetable or grain. We also need a reliable source of omega-3 fatty acids each day, which are found in cold-water fish, grass-fed meat, eggs from chickens fed flax meal or allowed to eat grass, crickets and other bugs, and flax and or hemp seeds It should be noted that the increase in life longevity is not the result of a change in nutrition, but despite it. New medical techniques, drugs, and technology, among other factors, are responsible for the development of an older population.

We must teach our nation, especially our children, about the critical importance of eating vegetables and fruit to maintain health and vitality. Universal health care and free medications only *treat* existing chronic diseases. That is important, but most conventional treatments only control the symptoms of disease. They usually don't reverse damage that has already been done. Nor can they prevent disease in the first place. If we want to restore health and vitality to the young and old, we must see the connection between what we eat and our health, so we know how to provide our bodies with all the building blocks necessary for healthy living.

Our grandmothers were right. We all need to be eating a hefty serving of greens and fruit with every meal. If we want a healthy nation with higher productivity and lower health care costs, we must take our collective DNA out of the trash heap and put it back in the black, nutritious Iowa soil. If we don't, no matter how many trillions we spend, our nation's health will continue to slide, and chronic diseases will continue to spread.

And I should know. I see it every day in my clinical practice. I am an internal medicine physician who works in a teaching hospital. I teach medical students and residents in the internal medicine primary care clinics. I am also the primary internal medicine physician for a traumatic brain injury clinic, which provides care for people suffering from traumatic brain injuries and the resulting post-traumatic stress disorder. For many years, when my patients and students asked about herbal medicines, food supplements, aromatherapy, and the like, I dismissed those "alternatives" as unproven, faddish therapies. That was before I was burdened with a progressive disease that could not be stopped, or even slowed, by the best evidence-based medicine.

I was diagnosed with relapsing-remitting multiple sclerosis in 2000. By 2003, my disease was reclassified as secondary progressive MS. Unfortunately, secondary progressive MS responds poorly to treatment. Patients usually experience a gradual loss of strength and endurance and they become progressively more disabled. As a physician, I was able to pick the finest doctors and have access to the best evidence-based care available. My doctors told me that functions lost to progressive MS would not return and that it would be best to try to prevent the loss of function and slow the disease if possible. I took chemotherapy drugs and other potent immune suppressants in an attempt to slow the rate of my decline, to no avail. By 2003, I needed a cane to walk. Not long after that, I needed an electric wheelchair almost all of the time. I walked less and less.

Once I was required to use a wheelchair, I studied the medical literature night after night while my family was asleep, trying to find other options for maintaining and possibly restoring my strength. Unfortunately, there were no clinical trials in which I could participate. I was left with the choice of remaining relatively passive, accepting the best care provided by the best people, or seeking some other alternative on my own.

I studied the basic science literature about MS, Parkinson's disease, Alzheimer's, and Huntington's to understand why brain cells died. I formulated my own theories about why disability occurs in MS. I designed a new treatment protocol for my disease and based my rehabilitation on my new theory, the idea that mitochondrial failure drove disability in MS. My treatment method produced remarkable increases in both my strength and my endurance. This experience has changed my life and how I practice medicine.

Despite the continuing work of doctors and scientists, the origin of MS remains unknown. The cause of the damage to the body of a person with MS has been identified as antibody complexes that destroy myelin, the protective covering surrounding nerves. This loss of myelin leads to breaks in the communication between the brain/spinal cord and the rest of the body, which results in weakness and/or disturbed sensations, including blindness, dizziness, and pain. There are probably several different pathways that lead to a person developing MS and the following factors and their interactions likely play a role in that development:

1. DNA (the genetic inheritance).
2. Infections.
3. Toxin exposures (eaten, inhaled, or absorbed through skin).
4. Micronutrient intake (food).
5. Hormonal balance.
6. Allergies or sensitization to food.
7. Stress level (physical, psychological, and spiritual).

Of these seven factors, the only one you cannot alter is the genes that you were born with. Some people's DNA is more laden with problems and tendencies toward disease than others. Similarly, beyond good health and hygiene practices and a healthy diet, which will contribute to a healthy immune system in the future, the toll taken on your body by past infections may or may not be reversible. But you *can* affect your health in tremendous ways by addressing the other five factors. This book aims to arm you with the knowledge to improve your health in every factor you can — which, in my case, led to dramatic improvement.

Most importantly, I will demonstrate that these seven factors affect more than just a possible MS diagnosis. All seven of them, some more so than others, play direct roles in the development of nearly *all* chronic disease, ranging from depression, learning disability, autism, diabetes, rheumatoid arthritis, and even Alzheimer's and Parkinson's.

For four years, I had to use a scooter or electric wheelchair whenever I left my office and needed two canes to walk even short distances. But now they sit, unused and dusty, in my office. I utilized a combination of nutrition and electrotherapy to restore my strength. Along the way, I felt like Paul on the way to Damascus. The old me was struck down and replaced by someone who sees the world of health and disease in an entirely new light. I am a different person, and a different physician. I now understand the profound connection between food and health. Medicines prescribed for MS, or any other disease, may control symptoms for a brief time, but if you want to be healed, you must eat the foods that your mitochondria and body need. Your DNA contains the wisdom to heal you. Unless doctors are treating an infection, we rarely provide true healing. Only you can provide your body with the building blocks for your cells so that they can do the work of restoring your health and vitality.

The health of our mitochondria affects the health of nearly every cell in the body. Because the diet of most Americans is severely lacking in the micronutrients needed for mitochondria to have optimal cellular function, our bodies can experience progressive damage to the mitochondria and our cells, leading to cells that do not function well, which in turn leads to progressive, lasting damage to our bodies. Many other diseases worsen because of sick mitochondria; diseases like asthma, chronic obstructive lung disease, hypertension, coronary artery disease, depression, obesity, bipolar disorder, and diabetes have all been shown to become worse as a result of mitochondrial stress and eventual failure. Mitochondrial failure drives the development of diabetes, heart disease, lung disease, heartburn from stomach acidity, Alzheimer's, Parkinson's, many psychiatric disorders, and multiple sclerosis. Improving the health of our mitochondria, by definition, improves the health of our cells. Healthy cells are necessary to have healthy organs; healthy organs lead to healthier bodies and restored vitality.

The drugs I prescribe to patients help control symptoms but they rarely restore normal physiology. Physicians rarely ensure their patients have the necessary building blocks for their cells to do the work of living. Although all physicians learn biochemistry in our first year of medical school, we do not learn to combine clinical nutrition with biochemistry. As a result, few physicians consider the nutrients that are needed for healthy functioning of one's mitochondria or one's brain.

Students typically study biology in high school and that curriculum does teach students about mitochondria. Unfortunately, our young people don't learn that the mitochondria within their bodies have specific requirements so that the substrates (or building blocks) can function well. Now, our grandparents didn't know about the technical aspects of this connection, either, but their diets reflected what they had learned over many centuries. Today, however, unhealthy food is marketed to us as cheap, quick, and safe, when, if analyzed carefully, none of these claims are true. It will take extensive educational efforts for us to return to a healthy diet and the wisdom of generations past.

In my practice, I spend a lot of time teaching my patients how the food they eat can lead either to a steady decline in health or steady restoration of vitality. I have organized this book in a similar fashion to how I teach patients in clinic, but I provide much more detail than I can cover in my clinics. I use basic metaphors to help the reader visualize what is happening in their cells as I explain the lives of our cells and our mitochondria, beginning with the basic biology of brain cells. I then review how the brain cells are wired to each other, how this wiring is insulated, and how the brain cells communicate with one another. Next, I talk about the marvelous chemical factory that exists in our cells through the release of neurotransmitter molecules. After that, I will show where the brain cell gets the energy to do all of its work. Finally, I explain the mitochondrial role in triggering cell death and the development of cancers.

The subsequent chapters discuss the role of specific micronutrients needed to support all of those important functions in the brain and the mitochondria. I also identify good food sources for these key micronutrients, so you can eat to specifically maximize the health of your mitochondria and brain. The Wahls Diet, rich in the micronutrients needed for healthy brains and healthy mitochondria, is explained next. To make these changes easier, I have provided recipes to help you get started on a nutrient-rich diet.

The final chapters review the scientific literature on the interventions I used on myself, which were important in my success to get me out of my wheelchair and back on my feet. I provide a theoretical framework for why my interventions have been so successful and discuss research on the biology of mitochondria, brain growth factors, the role of exercise, and the role of electrical therapy in MS.

In 2007, I read the design of a research study that was using electrical stimulation of muscles in people who were paralyzed; this inspired me to work with my physical therapist to use electrical stimulation on myself. Electrical stimulation of my muscles was an important part of the rehabilitation of my strength and stamina. This technology has been used for decades by athletes to grow larger, stronger muscles and to speed healing after injury. More recently, electrical stimulation has been used to help speed recovery of function after strokes, improve bladder control in patients with MS, decrease spasms in those with cerebral palsy, and improve the ability of patients disabled by severe heart disease to do the tasks of daily life.

Electrical stimulation, combined with intensive nutrition and daily exercise, allowed me to regain my strength and endurance more quickly than if I had relied on exercise alone. At this time, there is no published research that has used electrical stimulation of muscles to improve the strength and stamina of those with progressive MS. I have a research team studying whether the combination of intensive nutrition and electrical stimulation of muscles in others with progressive MS will lead to the improvement in function that I have been able to achieve. It is too early to specify what role electrical stimulation of muscles will have in the treatment of others who have become disabled by multiple sclerosis. Working with a physical therapist who is familiar with the use of electrical stimulation of muscles may be of extensive benefit. More research is needed to answer that question.

In the conclusion, I summarize the Wahls Diet and the simple things you can do to help heal your brain and your body, or at least slow the progression of a chronic disease, if one is affecting you. I also review what I think are the key research questions I'd like to answer regarding nutrition and traumatic brain injury, as well as the research questions I have about multiple sclerosis, nutrition, and electrical therapy of muscles.

Chapter Two
MITOCHONDRIA

Life exists because of controlled, reproducible biochemical reactions. Plants use chloroplasts to convert sunlight into energy in a process called photosynthesis. Animals cannot do this, so all animals, humans included, must consume food for energy. Mitochondria (singular: mitochondrion) are tiny subunits (organelles) inside our cells enclosed by a membrane. Eons ago, they may even have been separate from our animal ancestors, and joined with us to live as part of our cells for our benefit. They are, in brief, the power plants that keep our cells going and perform many of the functions that are absolutely critical to cellular processes, and therefore, our lives. Although they are not the "quarterback," that is, they are not the nucleus that holds the DNA, they are the engine of life.

Among other things, mitochondria metabolize, or detoxify, the poisons that get into our blood and, therefore, into our cells. These toxins can include excessive medicines, pesticides and toxins in our food and water, and pollutants in the air we breathe. Within the mitochondria there are a number of pathways in the electron-transport chain that change the chemical structure of poisonous compounds so that they can be safely excreted by the kidneys into urine or by the liver into bile.

Mitochondria also provide the signal to the cell to indicate that it is time to die. As a result of this signal, the cell allows a large amount of calcium to stream into the cell, causing cell death. It is important that our cells die at the appropriate time. Without that signal from the mitochondria, a cell becomes "immortal" and grows at the expense of everything else, becoming a cancerous tumor.

But above all, mitochondria should be thought of as the power plants that generate most of the energy our cells — and therefore our bodies and minds — need to function.

ATP

In humans and other animals, food energy is converted by the mitochondria into a substance called *adenosine tri-phosphate*, or ATP, which is stored for future use. ATP drives the creation of proteins, antibodies, cell walls, and new cells — in short, everything in our bodies. ATP is the currency of energy in every cell and, therefore, the currency of life. Without ATP, cells eventually die, and when too many cells die, the body dies.

Where in the cells is ATP made?

Cellular ATP is mostly produced by our mitochondria. While it is possible for some cells to make ATP without mitochondria, that method is inefficient and very wasteful. For that reason, our cells prefer to make ATP in the mitochondria.

The types of cells that require a lot of ATP to function have a lot of mitochondria. In humans, the highest concentration of mitochondria is found in the brain, followed by the retina, the heart, the tongue, the liver, and then muscles. This high concentration of mitochondria and great need for energy explains why the brain is so sensitive to deprivation of oxygen or glucose. When it is cut off from either substance, brain cells begin to die within a matter of minutes.

How exactly does the body make ATP?

Without oxygen, a cell can make two ATP molecules from one molecule of glucose (sugar). That is exactly what we do when we have to generate energy without oxygen (anaerobic metabolism), like when we sprint for short distances. However, if we pace ourselves so that we have a steady supply of oxygen and are using our aerobic (with oxygen) metabolism, our mitochondria can produce many more ATP molecules.

The Krebs cycle and the electron transport chain

If a cell must generate ATP without mitochondria, it can produce two ATP molecules per glucose molecule.[1] But with a healthy mitochondrion (singu-

---

1. See note at right.

lar form of mitochondria), a cell can make a total of 38 ATP molecules from one glucose molecule. Furthermore, depending on the energy needs of the cell, it can have hundreds, even thousands of mitochondria, churning out ATP for that particular cell. Brain cells, not surprisingly, have some of the highest concentrations of mitochondria per cell. It is therefore absolutely critical that we maintain mitochondrial health.

The mitochondria use specific substances that work as catalysts or co-factors to facilitate all of the various reactions necessary to generate the ATP. These co-factors are necessary to the process. Riboflavin (vitamin B2) is used to make FADH, and niacinamide (vitamin B3) is used to make NADH. Ubiquinone, also known as co-enzyme Q10, is another key co-factor in the electron transport chain. Thus, B vitamins and co-enzyme Q10 are important nutrients for healthy mitochondria.

Our mitochondria serve as a power plant for our cells and, as with every manufacturing process, some trash is left behind when the energy is manufactured. For mitochondria, the trash is something called free radicals, which have come into the national spotlight only recently. The mitochondria are a very efficient furnace, converting 97% of the energy stored in a glucose molecule to energy stored in ATP. If the mitochondria don't have enough B vitamins or co-enzyme Q, the mitochondria produce three to five times more of these free radicals and significantly less ATP.

Free Radicals
What happens to the free radicals that are generated as byproducts of ATP creation? They quickly look for material to combine with or oxidize. They will attack whatever is nearby, and the closest structure is the mitochondria. Not far away in the cell is the nuclear DNA, the genetic blueprints. If too much of a mitochondrion, is oxidized, then it can no longer generate ATP. Kill off too many mitochondria, and the cell will have a harder and harder time doing the work that is assigned to it. If the cellular DNA is at-

1. By utilizing a process of chemical reactions called the Krebs cycle within the mitochondria, four ATP molecules are generated along with six NADH (*niacinamide adenosine dinucleotide*) and two FADH (*flavin adenosine dinucleotide*) molecules. The FADH and NADH molecules are processed through a number of chemical reactions in the electron transport chain within the mitochondria. They facilitate the passage of electrons from one compound to another. In so doing, they allow the cell to make thirty-four more ATP molecules.

tacked by free radicals and oxidized, the cell's instruction manual will become damaged and the cell will be unable to function correctly. The result is premature aging and, eventually, far worse.

More and more chronic diseases are being discovered to be caused by damage from free radicals or are accelerated by damage caused by free radicals. Excess free radical damage can also cause the mitochondria to send a message to the cell nucleus (the "brain" of the cell) to initiate the pre-programmed cell death. That leads to premature aging. Worse yet, excess free radical damage to cell DNA can make the cell think it *never* has to die. Once that happens, the cell has become "immortal" and grows at the expense of everything else. We call that cancer.

The body's defense against free radicals is intracellular antioxidants. With an abundant supply of antioxidants in the mitochondria, the free radicals are quickly neutralized. So, where do we get these important antioxidants? The richest source of antioxidants comes from the richly colored vegetables and fruits. Purple, black, blue, red, orange, yellow, and green vegetables and fruits all have different supporting roles for our mitochondria, because those colors represent different kinds and levels of antioxidants. This is why eating a variety of colors each day is so beneficial, and so important, for you.

Studies have demonstrated that the people who the eat the highest amounts of greens and vegetables in the cabbage family, which are incredibly rich in B vitamins and antioxidants, have the lowest rates of degenerative diseases, such as macular degeneration of the retina, cataracts, atherosclerosis, rheumatoid arthritis, diabetes, or obesity. Multiple epidemiologic studies have shown that people who eat the highest levels of fruits and green vegetables have the lowest risk for *all forms* of cancer. Similarly, there are fewer age-related health problems for people with diets high in the B vitamins and antioxidants.

Mitochondria in Cell Life and Death
The mitochondria have many other roles in the cell in addition to energy generation. They remove toxins from the bloodstream, including toxins from medications, pesticides, and herbicide residues in our food.

As science has improved our understanding of the interactions between mitochondria, oxidative stress, and disease, we can now see that mitochondrial health is linked to chronic disease. In diabetes, obesity, excessive cholesterol levels, rheumatoid arthritis, asthma, and multiple sclerosis,

MITOCHONDRIA IN CELL LIFE AND DEATH

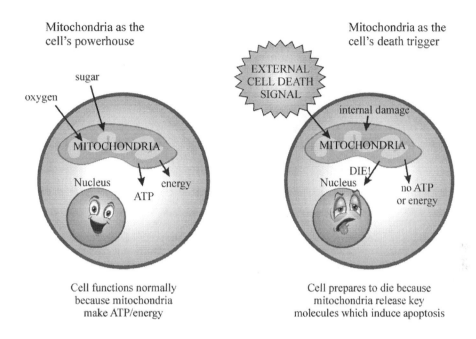

Mitochondria as the
cell's powerhouse

Mitochondria as the
cell's death trigger

EXTERNAL
CELL DEATH
SIGNAL

oxygen

sugar

internal damage

MITOCHONDRIA

MITOCHONDRIA

DIE!

Nucleus

energy

Nucleus

no ATP
or energy

ATP

Cell functions normally
because mitochondria
make ATP/energy

Cell prepares to die because
mitochondria release key
molecules which induce apoptosis

oxidative stress is a major contributing factor to accelerating the disease's progress.

The level of intracellular vitamins and antioxidants depends almost exclusively upon the food we eat. Diets rich in simple sugars and carbohydrates, but lacking in vegetables and fruits, have very few minerals, vitamins, or antioxidants. As such, people who eat micronutrient *poor* diets leave their cells and mitochondria at risk for damage from free radicals. A lifetime of exposure to these free radicals accelerates the aging processes and increases the risk of cancers of all types, autoimmune disease, and other degenerative diseases. This is why diets that are rich in vegetables, particularly greens, have been shown in study after study to lower the risk of malignancies, macular degeneration, cataracts, Alzheimer's, and other degenerative diseases.

In summary, mitochondria are important to the healthy functioning of the cell, and therefore the body. Mitochondria are tiny chemical power plants responsible for the efficient conversion of the energy in food to a form of energy (ATP) that the cell needs to function. Like all chemical plants, a small amount of trash, free radicals, is made during the process of ATP production. Antioxidants are used by the mitochondria to safely remove free radicals before the free radicals can damage the cell. Antioxidants are found in fruits and vegetables. Mitochondria have two other important functions. They are responsible for telling the cell when it is time to die (programmed cell death) and it is the mitochondria that remove the toxins from the body.

Chapter Three
CELLULAR FUNCTION AND BRAIN HEALTH

Each of us has approximately one billion brain cells. Each brain cell, taken alone, is essentially worthless. But collectively, when all of our brain's cells are richly connected and talking to each other, our brains have judgment, experience, and, hopefully, some accumulated wisdom. The brain requires vast amounts of energy in the form of ATP to function properly. This chapter will summarize important nutritional concepts as they relate to brain health. Some of the key functions of the brain cells include wiring the brains cells to one another, building insulation (myelin) around the wiring (dendrites and axons), and communicating with each other through the release of neurotransmitters. Because the brain cells do so much work, they need a lot of ATP, and without ATP, the brain cells begin to die very quickly. This is why mitochondria have such a key role in brain health. I will discuss each of these functions briefly and identify some of the important nutrients that support the brain's ability to complete these tasks.

Mitochondria in the Brain

The brain and the retinas of the eyes have the greatest need for cellular energy in order to do their work. Our brains continually take in sensory data from our eyes, ears, tongue, nose, and skin. The retina in the eye provides the brain with a continuous motion picture, transmitting bits of information to the brain constantly. We interpret the stream of data in the context of all our prior experiences, to know whether we are safe or in danger. All of that takes energy, so it should be no surprise that our brains and retinas have the most mitochondria per cell and that they are utterly dependent upon an immediate supply of both oxygen and glucose. Lose access to either one, and the mitochondria cannot produce ATP, thus cells in the brain and retina quickly begin to die.

These chemical reactions in the mitochondria—the creation of energy, timing of cell death, and detoxification of the cells—are dependent upon a rich supply of B vitamins, co-enzyme Q, iodine, and antioxidants from colorful fruits and vegetables. Unfortunately, the majority of Americans eat less than two cups of vegetables and fruit each day. Fewer eat any organ meats, also an excellent supply of sulfur and many B vitamins and other micronutrients important to brain health. The result is that most Americans do not sufficiently supply their mitochondria with proper nutrition. Less ATP is created, causing increasingly inefficient mitochondria, and a brain that is less able to repair damage or respond to any medications that are trying to increase or decrease neurotransmitters.

Axons and Dendrites

The brain creates billions of connections between the brain cells. These connections are called *axons* and *dendrites*, and energy is needed to build and maintain them. The brain cells transmit information down the axons and dendrites to the next brain cell in the line of communication. The brain is similar to an electrical grid and to keep the information flowing quickly and accurately, the grid wiring needs insulation. Without insulation, called *myelin*, the flow of information along these electrical pathways slows down, can jump to other wires, and send the information to the wrong areas. This is what happens in MS. The insulation in the brain becomes thin and absent in some places, and as a result, information is sometimes unable to reach its proper destination. If motor nerves are affected, problems with coordination and weakness occur; problems with pain, vision, or balance are linked to damage to the sensory nerve pathways.

Myelin and Cell Membranes

How does the brain cell make the insulation needed to keep the information flow secure? Like just about everything else, mitochondria are the manufacturers. *Glial cells* are special brain cells that wrap around the axons and dendrites of the brain cells. Glial cells can repair areas where myelin has been damaged if they have enough ATP and the building blocks for myelin. Omega-3 fatty acids are the key building blocks for myelin. The brain must also have an adequate supply of B vitamins, particularly thiamin (vitamin B1) and cobolamin (vitamin B12). Because the standard Western diet has so few fruits and vegetables, many of us are at risk of having inadequate levels of multiple B vitamins.[16-18] Furthermore, the vast majority of Americans eat diets that have very few omega-3 fatty acids.[19,20] This can partly be attributed to not eating much fish, but most Americans also eat meat and eggs from animals that are fed and fattened on corn, which is very rich in omega-6 fatty acids and has minimal omega-3 fatty acids.

Omega-6 fatty acids are important in the creation of many key molecules in our bodies. However, a diet too rich in omega-6 fatty acids alters certain molecular pathways, or rewires the grid, causing misinformation and making the body generate more inflammation. On the other hand, diets rich in omega-3 fatty acids lower the level of inflammation molecules in the body and in the brain. A higher number of inflammation molecules are believed to worsen autoimmune diseases of all types, including MS.

For many Americans, the ratio of omega-6 to omega-3 fatty acids in our diet is 30 to 1. For coastal communities with a seafood-based diet, the ratio is 3 to 1. Notably, in communities with seafood-based diets, there is a 10- to 100-fold lower incidence of diseases, such as multiple sclerosis and mental health diagnoses, as compared to populations that eat land-based diets, with an omega-3 to omega-6 ratio of 15 to 1 or greater.

Neurotransmitters
The brain uses molecules called neurotransmitters as signals to communicate between one nerve cell and another. A variety of small molecules, many of them amino acids, fulfill this communication role. When the nerve cell receives a signal from another nerve cell or sensory receptor, the signal goes along the length of the dendrite, back to the cell body, and down the axon, which reaches to the next brain cell, where depolarization occurs. Depolarization is an electrical change that needs to happen in order for the message to be transmitted. If there is plenty of myelin, the depolarization is fast and transmission time is short. If the myelin is gone, the information can still be transmitted, but much more slowly, as it requires the use of an increased number of sodium channels. Once the information has been transmitted down the length of the nerve, molecules called neurotransmitters must be released and picked up by the brain cell on the pathway to continue the communication process.

MS patients experience acute symptoms in the form of a relapse when these myelin gaps cause a break in transmission, as I have experienced in my own life. When the nerve finally adds more sodium channels and can transmit information again, the symptoms decline and the patient has a remission of symptoms. MS patients also typically experience a variety of neurotransmitter imbalances, including *glutamate, gamma amino butyric acid* (GABA), *serotonin*, and, to a lesser extent, *norepinephrine*.

The most damaging problem with neurotransmitters may be the excessive levels of glutamate coupled with too much stimulation of the *N methyl D aspartate*, or NMDA, receptor.[21,22] Glutamate is important to both learning and shortening response times to specific stimuli or tasks. However, when the amount of glutamate becomes excessive, the brain cell can become over-stimulated, leading to intracellular stress and even, sometimes, early death of the brain cell. Toxic amounts of glutamate are seen in circumstances with chronic physical pain, increased stiffness, and seizures.[23] High glutamate levels are believed to play a role in anxiety, depression, obsessive-compulsive disorders, and possibly other psychiatric disorders.[24] Two common food additives increase the brain levels of glutamate.[25-27] One is monosodium glutamate (MSG), a flavor enhancer often found in restaurant food, particularly Chinese cooking. The other additive is aspartame (NutraSweet®), which is a sweetener commonly found in diet beverages of all types. Some individuals have headaches if they eat anything with either MSG or NutraSweet®. Eliminating these from your diet is prudent if you are suffering from any neurological or psychiatric symptoms.

Fortunately, the brain has a way to rebalance glutamate levels. In the brain, *gamma amino butyric acid* (GABA) and glutamate balance each other out. GABA is one of the most important inhibitory neurotransmitters, and it allows the body to have coordinated, fluid movements, and helps control impulsive behavior. Some believe it is an important factor in mood disorders, including obsessive-compulsive disorder, depression, and anxiety.[28,29] As an inhibitory neurotransmitter, GABA helps with calming and quieting both physical and mental pain and distress.[30-32] For someone experiencing excessive pain, muscle stiffness, or persisting emotional distress, the brain levels of GABA are likely too low. Anxiety, pain, and irritability are typically increased.

The level of GABA in the brain can be manipulated by certain drugs, such as *Gabapentin* and *baclofen*, which are often used to treat MS symptoms. They both stimulate the release of GABA. Gabapentin is often used to treat pain related to MS nerve damage. Baclofen is used to treat the stiffness or increased muscle tone due to damage by MS to the nerves leading to the muscles.

GABA can also be manipulated by adding specific nutrients to the diet.[33,34] You can't simply increase your level of GABA by eating it, because it does not cross the blood-brain barrier. But you can increase your consumption of nutrients your brain uses to make GABA, such as organic sulfur, which comes from amino acids like *N-acetyl cysteine, methionine*, and *taurine*. *Glutathione* is very important to the generation of GABA because the brain cells also use glutathione to recycle and regenerate the GABA.[35] Because the generation of neurotransmitters is dependent on diets rich in specific amino acids, the amount of organic sulfur in your diet will either make it very difficult, or relatively easy, for your brain to make and maintain the desired levels of GABA.

Two other neurotransmitters that may be affected by MS include serotonin and norepinephrine.[35,36] Low levels of serotonin lead to depression, irritability, and aggression. Medications are often given to boost the levels of serotonin or the brain cells' responsiveness to serotonin. Another transmitter that can become problematic is norepinephrine, which is secreted by the adrenal glands and by the brain in response to stress. Too much norepinephrine leads to problems focusing, an inability to tune out distractions, and increased anxiety.

Food Sensitivities
There is another, often overlooked, problem that can interfere with brain-cell function. Celiac disease, which is essentially an allergy to gluten, is associated with mood issues, learning problems, fatigue, weakness, and MS-like symptoms.[35,37,38] Over the last generation, celiac disease has occurred more frequently in both children and adults. Celiac disease is a well-described entity in which the body is allergic to the protein gluten in wheat. As a result, antibodies are made that attack the lining of the gut and, in some cases, other structures in the body. Not all patients report diarrhea or abdominal complaints. Patients with celiac disease often have a long history of vague, poorly explained psychological or neurological symptoms with or without abdominal symptoms. Because celiac disease is a great masquerader with innumerable vague symptoms that are not related to the gut, it can often takes years to come to a diagnosis.

For anyone with neurological issues or mental health issues, it may be worthwhile to explore with your medical providers the possibility of food allergies. In addition to wheat, it is possible to be sensitive to other foods that lead to a "leaky gut," which allows compounds into the body that a healthy gut would not permit.[39-41] This leakiness increases the risk of developing food allergies and the development of antibodies toward the offending food(s), and multiple vague symptoms.

Because it can take 72 hours for symptoms to occur, it can be challenging to sort out what foods may be causing which symptoms. There are a variety of books now available that are about food sensitivities and elimination diets used to help identify the offending foods. See the appendix for a graphic depicting how unrecognized food allergies may cause or worsen autoimmune and other chronic disease problems.

Books and Other Resources
Additional information on diet, micronutrients, cellular function, and health can be found in such books as *Eat to Live* and *Eat for Health*, both by Dr. Joel Fuhrman, *The Whole Life Nutrition Cookbook* by Tom Malterre and Alisisa Segersten, and *The World's Healthiest Foods* by George Mateljan. Another excellent source of information on micronutrients can be found at the Linus Pauling Institute for Micronutrients at Oregon State University: **http://lpi.oregonstate.edu/**.

The Institute of Functional Medicine is a medical organization dedicated to teaching healthcare providers how to manage chronic, complex medical problems, such as multiple sclerosis, chronic fatigue syndrome, multiple chemical sensitivities, and more. It teaches physicians, nutritionists, and others about functional clinical nutrition, and the role that problems with poor nutrition, excessive toxic load, inflammation, hormone imbalance, chronic infections, and spiritual disequilibrium have in driving disease. It has a number of excellent texts and seminars on the integration of nutrition, cellular function, disease, and health. Their Web site is **http://www. functionalmedicine.org/**. See the appendix for a graphic that depicts how Functional Medicine differs from Conventional Medicine. More information can be found at that Web site. You will also find listings for the names of health care providers in your area that have received training in functional medicine. If you have a complex, chronic health problem that conventional doctors are not solving, I recommend you investigate finding a health care provider that has received training from the Institute of Functional Medicine.

The Center for Mind-Body Medicine provides information for healthcare professionals and the lay public on nutrition and the use of food to assist with the prevention and healing of chronic disease. Their Web site is **http:// www.cmbm.org/.**

Chapter Four
MICRONUTRIENTS, SUPPLEMENTS, AND FOOD SOURCES

This chapter explores the impact of micronutrients (i.e., the vitamins, minerals, and essential fats) on your brain cells and on your overall health. I will also discuss specific strategies to maximize these key micronutrients in your diet. Although there is considerable interest in the genetic causes of disease, I have found that environmental factors, particularly the micronutrient content of the diet, are the primary cause of most chronic diseases. It is the deficient diet that turns genes off and on, often leading to activation of genes associated with cleft lip, crooked teeth, learning disabilities, diabetes, obesity, and heart disease.

Dr. Weston Price, a dentist, analyzed the diets of 14 different primitive peoples from five continents in the early twentieth century. Because there are very few cultures now that have not been Westernized, researchers would have a very difficult time conducting a similar type of study today. He studied individuals who were still eating the traditional foods for that culture, and the first and second generation of individuals who had adopted a Westernized diet. His team analyzed the nutritional contents of the primitive and Westernized diets, and conducted physical assessments, mental assessments, dental x-rays, and assessments of bone densities. His book *Nutrition and Physical Degeneration* was first published in 1936.

His findings demonstrated that there was considerable variation in the local foodstuffs, as the diets accommodated what was locally available. In spite of the variation, the primitive diets consistently were very rich in vitamins, minerals, and omega-3 fatty acids. The Westernized diets were consistently lacking in vitamins, minerals, and omega-3 fatty acids. The individuals who were eating traditional, primitive diets had straight teeth without cavities, while the individuals with a Westernized diet had crooked teeth filled with cavities. Furthermore, the individuals eating a primitive diet had superior physical and mental assessments, as compared to those who ate a Westernized diet.

His conclusion was that lack of micronutrients led to physical degeneration. He believed that diets deficient in micronutrients activated certain genes, which led to stunted growth of the mid-face, decreased intelligence, and emotional instability, as well as lower mineral content in bones and lower muscle mass. More recent studies have confirmed diets deficient in omega-3 fatty acids are associated with numerous health and dental problems, including mal-aligned teeth and higher rates of orthodontia dental work, learning disabilities, depression, and excessive aggression. Diets lower in fruits and vegetables (antioxidants) are associated with higher rates of cancers, cataracts, macular degeneration, diabetes, high blood pressures, heart disease, and autoimmune diseases like multiple sclerosis. It has been empirically proven that what we do and do not eat affects the functions of our cells and, therefore, our overall health.

Many authors have studied primitive diets, or "Paleolithic diets," concluding that traditional diets were much richer in vitamins, minerals, essential fatty acids, and other important phytonutrients (plant-based nutrients) and were associated with greater health.[42-57] The standard American diet leaves over 90% of Americans over the age of two with inadequate intake of essential fats, vitamins, and minerals, due to its emphasis on white flour, sugar, high-fructose corn syrup, seeds high in omega-6 fats instead of greens high in omega-3 fats, and animals fed seeds (like corn) instead of grass. This diet is strongly associated with autoimmune and chronic degenerative disease and a return to the Paleolithic diet reduces many of the symptoms of our modern autoimmune and chronic degenerative diseases.[44,45,58-60] Additionally, many modern diets are low in iodine and trace minerals,[61-66] which have significant implications for health of our brains and our mitochondria. What we have learned from those studies is that people can eat a wide variety of foodstuffs and retain our health. There were some foods that were consistently associated with poor dental, mental, and physical health. Those were sugar, white flour, white potatoes, and a grain-rich diet—the mainstay of the American diet. No wonder we are progressively less well.

General Diet Recommendations:
If you want optimal health, it is critical to maximize the micronutrients in your diet. Not only do most Americans eat barely two cups of fruits and vegetables per day, they eat a relatively narrow range of these foods. Such diets do not provide optimal nutrition for the brain. In the next paragraphs I will describe an optimal diet for brain health.

Eat a wide variety of fruits and vegetables. Include red, blue, purple, yellow, and green fruits and vegetables. Gradually increase the number of servings per day, with a goal of at least nine cups of vegetables and fruits per day. Three cups should be dark green (spinach, Swiss chard, or mustard greens) or from the cruciferous (cabbage, kale, collards, broccoli) family, three cups should be intensely colored (red, orange, blue, purple, black), and three cups should be from others. Do *not* count white potatoes, corn, rice, or grain in the nine cups of vegetables and fruit. You can eat them, but do so after having achieved nine cups of vegetables and fruit first. Include some mushrooms, nutritional yeast, and nuts or seeds in your diet daily, if possible. Take in more minerals through the consumption of seaweed, dried kelp, and/or brewer's yeast.

Eat more omega-3-rich foods. These are green leaves and animals that feed on green leaves. It also includes wild fish, because the bottom of the fish food chain is green algae, rich in omega-3 fats. (Be sure your fish is low in mercury, however.) An excellent guide to low mercury fish can be found at **http://www.nrdc.org/health/effects/mercury/ guide.asp**. Eat meat from grass-fed animals and omega-3-enriched eggs from chickens that have been fed flax meal or that have been allowed free range to eat bugs, crickets, and greens. Other options for omega-3 fatty acids include fish oil, flax oil, and hemp oil. One to two tablespoons of flax or hemp oil daily is comparable to two to four grams of fish oil. Note that if you are taking blood thinners, such as coumadin, aspirin, or other medicines to thin your blood, taking additional fish oil increases the risk of bleeding complications. Therefore, it is important to speak with your personal physician prior to starting fish oil or any vitamins or mineral supplements. Eat organ meats once a week, because they are a tremendous source of B vitamins and important mitochondrial nutrients.

Supplements

Many people ask me if they can just take supplements and not change their diets. That doesn't work. There are likely hundreds, if not thousands, of other key micronutrients, which have not yet been identified but are present in food that is rich in micronutrients. While I use several supplements to boost the micronutrient intake for my mitochondria, I also consume three to six cups (600 grams) of cruciferous vegetables and 300 grams of deeply pigmented fruit and/or vegetables each day, and add seaweed to my soups and vegetables for the iodine and trace minerals. Keep in mind that having a plateful of kale (about 300 to 600 grams) is the equivalent of taking hundreds of capsules of sulfur-based amino acids. The food we eat has a more powerful effect than taking supplements. Taking a few pills containing the sulfur-based amino acids, while they may be helpful, are simply not as effective as eating a plateful of greens. Eating more non-starchy vegetables, colored fruits, nuts, and seeds can provide more amino acids, minerals, vitamins, and other essential phytonutrients than taking specific supplements each day.

I am often asked about the use of various herbal medicines to boost brain health. Although some of the herbal medicines have been used for thousands of years and are natural, the use of supplements and herbal medicines is not without hazard. First, one has to be concerned about the country of origin, because there have been reports of contaminants and heavy metals in some products. Secondly, research may not be available to support the claims made by the manufacturers of the supplements. The science is often incomplete in verifying whether the claimed benefits of various supplements and herbal products really do occur in the people taking them.

It is useful to look to third-party organizations and the National Institute of Health (NIH) for unbiased information about the helpfulness of supplements. An organization called Consumer Labs tests the purity of supplements and posts their results online at **http://www.consumerlab.com/**. Another way to have confidence in the purity of the vitamins and supplements that you purchase is to look the seal that indicates the manufacturer has been inspected by a third party in terms of product purity and is compliant with of Good Manufacturing Practices.

The NIH has a department called the National Center for Complementary and Alternative Medicine, with an active research program focused on learning more about the benefits and risks of such therapies. They provide consumer hotlines for the public and a large library of information about supplements and herbal medicines. Their Web site is **http://nccam.nih. gov/**.

I have provided a list of the specific nutrients that I have used. However, what I use may or may not be appropriate for anyone else, given each person's unique health issues. It is therefore important to talk to your pharmacist and your physicians about any supplements you wish to try before taking them. Your unique circumstances may render some of these supplements unhelpful, or possibly even harmful. In the appendix is a chart summarizing the nutrients, good sources in food, and the function of that nutrient in the brain.

Food has distinct advantages over supplements. The micronutrients in food are generally more readily able to be used by your body, and it is much less likely that you can absorb toxic levels of the micronutrient in question. Furthermore, you also have the benefit of absorbing the hundreds, if not thousands, of other micronutrients that our bodies need, but have not yet been classified by modern science.

The list of micronutrients and their food sources should help guide you in selecting a diet that provides the most nutrients possible for your mito-chondria and your brain. Supplements are sometimes helpful, particularly for those who have a neurological or psychiatric disorder, or a total-body deficit of particular nutrients due to a history of limited intake of vegeta-bles, fruits, and/or seafood. I do think that using a probiotic supplement, which is the "friendly" gut bacteria for the colon in capsule form, helps to reintroduce the beneficial bacteria into one's colon. An alternative strategy to introduce friendly bacteria into the colon is eating fermented foods, such as pickles and sauerkraut. The bacteria in our colon can either produce useful vitamins and compounds that we absorb through the colon wall or produce chemicals that are toxic to us. Because of the common use of an-tibiotics in the meat supply, even if you rarely take antibiotics, it is likely that the bacteria living in your gut have been altered. By taking probiotics you are reintroducing helpful bacteria and displacing the unhealthy ones.

Diets that are high in grains, carbohydrates, and sugars affect which types of bacteria can thrive in the colon. One may have bacteria living in one's colon that are not causing an infection, but are generating inflamma-tory molecules that lead to activation of arthritis. Thus, even in the absence of gluten sensitivity, taking a probiotic and minimizing the consumption of grain and other carbohydrates may be an important strategy in reducing inflammation in the body.

Micronutrients and Cellular Function

Again, in general, eating generous amounts of a food source of nutrients is better for you because there are many more micronutrients in real food than there are in supplements. Likely there are hundreds, if not thousands, of important micronutrients, which help our bodies function well, that we have yet to discover. In addition, we can often absorb and utilize the nutrients more effectively when they are in food.

The following briefly summarizes the benefits of each micronutrient, a few of its important functions in the body, doses that have been suggested as safe by other experts, and some good food sources for that nutrient. Also listed are herbal medicines that have studies to support their utility in supporting brain health.

Micronutrients for Cell Membrane and Myelin

Optimal cell membrane function requires avoidance of trans-fats (i.e., vegetable oil fats that have been partially hydrogenated to make them solid at room temperature) and the ingestion of omega-3 fatty acids. Omega-3 fatty acids are an essential part of healthy, fluid cell membranes. Fish oil is the most effective way to increase your levels of two fatty acids, EPA (*eicosopentanoic acid*) and DHA (*docosohexanoic acid*). The best source is three or more servings per week of cold-water fish, such as wild salmon, mackerel, or tuna. Many grocers now carry, in their organic food section, eggs from chickens that have been fed flax meal. These are labeled either as Omega-3-enriched eggs or DHA eggs.

Meat from corn-fed animals has a very low amount of omega-3 fatty acids; the majority of commercial meat in the U.S is corn-fed, not free-range or grass-fed, which is one reason why most Americans have such low intake of this important nutrient. Grass-fed animals have a more balanced amount of omega-3 fatty acids. There are some niche farmers who raise grass-fed cattle, sheep, and free-range chickens. Checking with a local farmers' market or food co-op is usually an effective way to find meat that is from grass-fed animals rather than corn-fed animals.

The level of HDL (good cholesterol) in the body tends to mirror the ratio of omega-3 to omega-6 fatty acids. The lower the level of omega-3 in your body and your brain, the lower the HDL level tends to be. Increasing the amount of omega-3 fatty acids in the diet will generally boost the HDL level, which should be, at minimum, above forty mg/ dl and, if possible, above sixty. If you use fish oil, after checking with your doctor, start by taking one capsule and work up gradually over several weeks to two to four per day. For those who cannot tolerate fish oil, flax or hemp oil are possible alternatives. Since your body can convert ten percent of flax oil into omega-3 fatty acids for your cell membranes, you need more flax oil than fish oil. Start with one teaspoon per day and work gradually up to one to two tablespoons. Eggs high in DHA, hemp-seed oil, and hemp seed butter are other good sources of omega-3 fatty acids.

Because the bacteria in your colon have to get used to the addition of omega-3 fatty acids to your diet, a few people experience a lot of bloating and gas when first adding fish oil or flax oil to their diet. If that is a problem for you, a probiotic can be taken for several weeks to help your digestive system get used to the new diet.

Micronutrients for Mitochondria

Without the ATP molecules generated by the mitochondria, it becomes difficult for the cell to carry out the tasks it is supposed to do, such as making neurotransmitters and antibodies, or repairing cellular damage from everyday life. The brain and eye have the highest number of mitochondria per cell, followed by the heart and tongue. Important co-factors necessary for generation of ATP include B vitamins and co-enzyme Q.

When the mitochondria make ATP, a small amount of toxic free radicals are generated. Antioxidants from fruits and vegetables make it easier for the mitochondria to neutralize the free radicals. Particularly potent intracellular antioxidants are *glutathione, Lipoic acid, L Carnitine*, and *Resveratrol. Creatine phosphate* is helpful because it helps facilitate the generation of ATP. In the next section I'll discuss each micronutrient's main contribution to brain health and good food sources in more detail.

Vitamins

As I here describe some of the functions of vitamins as they relate to brain function, keep in mind it is best to have your personal physician monitor the use of supplements, including vitamins. Some physicians have advocated high doses of vitamin B1 (thiamin) for people with degenerative brain conditions like Parkinson's, Alzheimer's, and multiple sclerosis.[67] Dr. Frederich R. Klenner and Dr. H. T. Mount, have separately reported success using nutritional approaches to treat MS, based upon a liver extract, which is a potent source of B vitamins.[68,69] They believe that high doses of B1, B2 (riboflavin), B3 (niacinamide), and B12 (cobolamin) were beneficial for those suffering from poor brain health. Inadequate intake of B vitamins has been associated with cognitive decline and multiple progressive causes of brain decline and neurodegeneration.[70-77] Ensuring adequate intake of micronutrients is therefore very important to brain health.

Thiamin (Vitamin B1)

Thiamin supports mitochondrial function in the brain. Without thiamin, it is more difficult for mitochondria to generate ATP molecules. Thiamin is also an important co-factor, along with vitamin B12, in helping the brain cells make myelin to insulate the nerve.

Ensuring plenty of thiamin in one's diet is important for anyone with MS. Thiamin is secreted by the kidneys and is generally not stored in the body. It is important to have a steady supply in your diet. Good food sources include sunflower seeds, mushrooms, yeast, spinach, sunflower seeds, tuna, tomatoes, asparagus, black beans, cabbage, and kale.

- How much thiamin can I safely take each day?

Because the body can easily rid itself of the excess thiamin through the kidneys, an upper limit for safe amount of thiamin has not been established. Physicians have used thiamin to treat alcohol-related brain damage, because excessive alcohol use can cause severe thiamin deficiency. As a result, alcoholics can develop brain damage causing problems with memory, coordination, balance, and problems with heart failure. The typical dose of thiamine given to alcoholics experiencing thiamine deficiency is 100 mg per day. Thus, up to 100 mg of thiamin each day would generally be safe.

Riboflavin (Vitamin B2)

Riboflavin is part of the FADH complex of enzymes used by the mitochondria to convert the energy stored in food to the energy stored in ATP, which the cells can use for day-to-day functions. It is also a critical nutrient for the elimination of toxins. Riboflavin deficiency has been associated with poor mitochondrial health and increased oxidative stress. Riboflavin deficiency is rarely found in isolation, but it occurs frequently in combination with deficiencies of other water-soluble vitamins. Most foods derived from plants or animals contain at least small quantities of riboflavin. Good sources in food include almonds, fish, broccoli, and asparagus.

- How much riboflavin can I safely take each day?

A dose of 200 milligrams a day of riboflavin has been used successfully to treat both migraine and tension headaches. No upper limit of daily intake has been identified, thus supplemental riboflavin is likely to be well tolerated.

Niacinamide (Vitamin B3)

Niacinamide is an important nutrient for brain health. It is a key nutrient for mitochondria, which are the powerhouse for brain cells. The mitochondria convert the energy that is stored in sugar into the energy the cell can use to do its work in the form of ATP. An ample supply of niacinamide makes the generation of ATP more efficient and reduces the level of free radicals. The best food sources are wheat germ, mushrooms, organ meats, tuna, and salmon.

Vitamin B3, or niacinamide, has been shown to be beneficial in a number of autoimmune diseases. Almost fifty years ago, Dr. William Kaufman used niacinamide to successfully reduce symptoms and improve function in patients with rheumatoid arthritis.[78] Twenty years ago, Dr. Kazuya Yamada reported that niacinamide reduces the severity of and can even reverse early type 1 diabetes in mice.[79-82] In 2006, Dr. Shinjiro Kaneko reported that using niacinamide was effective in preventing and reducing the severity of existing disease in mice with multiple sclerosis.[83] However, studies have not been published about humans using niacinamide to treat or prevent MS.

- How much niacinamide can I safely take each day?

Studies have shown that liver problems can occur with high doses of supplemental niacin. In 1998, the Institute of Medicine at the National Academy of Sciences set a tolerable upper intake limit (UL) for niacin of 35 milligrams. This UL applies to men and women nineteen or older, and is limited to niacin that is obtained from supplements and/or fortified foods. The niacin version of B3 has been used in doses between 500 and 3000 mg under the supervision of a physician for the treatment of high cholesterol and rheumatoid arthritis. However, because of the potential for problems with high doses (anything over 500 mg), it is *very important* to have a physician monitor liver function with blood tests to ensure no damage is occurring as a result of the higher dose. Even though it is easily available as an over-the-counter supplement, it is important to respect this important vitamin's potential to cause damage to the liver at doses above 500 mg per day.

Pyridoxine (Vitamin B6)

The role of pyridoxine involves many aspects of neurological activity. It is very important in making many neurotransmitters, including serotonin and GABA. A long list of prescription medications has been linked to depletion of the body's pyridoxine. These medications include many drugs that patients with MS are likely to take: birth control pills and oral estrogens, diuretics, anti-seizure drugs (often prescribed for pain control), and other drugs, such as asthma medications and antibiotics.

Good food sources for pyridoxine include garlic, tuna, cauliflower, mustard greens, bananas, celery, cabbage, crimini mushrooms, asparagus, broccoli, kale, collard greens, Brussels sprouts, cod, and chard.

- How much pyridoxine can I safely take each day?

Taking supplemental pyridoxine is not without risk. Imbalances in nervous system activity have been shown to result from high doses of pyridoxine. The National Academy of Sciences has set a tolerable UL of 100 mg for adults 19 years and older, largely based on the issue of potential neurotoxicity for people who metabolize pyridoxine more slowly.

Cobolamin (vitamin B12)

The body requires cobolamin in order to make hemoglobin (the oxygen-carrying portion of our red blood cells). It is also necessary, along with thiamin, for brain cells to effectively make myelin. We cannot make B12, but must consume it in our diet. Good food sources include liver, venison, shrimp, scallops, salmon, and beef. Vegetarians can get some B12 from sea plants (like kelp), algae (like spirulina), yeasts (like brewer's yeast), and fermented plant foods (like tempeh, miso, or tofu). However, because of the risk of inadequate levels of B12, vegetarians are strongly advised to take supplemental B12. The absorption of B12 is also dependent on something called *intrinsic factor*, which must be made in the stomach. People with stomach problems, such as gastritis, and individuals older than 60 years are at much greater risk of B12 deficiency.

Many neurologists advise their MS patients take the type of B12 supplement that can be absorbed under the tongue. That eliminates the need for intrinsic factor to absorb the B12. Anemia as a result of low B12 levels is thought to affect two percent of people over the age of sixty. Some drugs that are commonly prescribed also diminish the body's supply of vitamin B12, including anticonvulsants, antihypertensive medication, cholesterol-lowering drugs, and potassium replacements. In addition, it may be preferable for up to 20% of Americans to take the form of B12 called methylcobolamin, because they have problems with their methylation enzymes (see Toxicology chapter).

• How much cobolamin can I safely take each day?
When the National Academy of Sciences established its current UL for the B complex vitamins in 1998, it did not establish a UL for vitamin B12. Even long-term studies, in which subjects have taken 1,000 micrograms (mcg) of the vitamin every day for five years, have revealed no toxic effects.

Folic Acid

Folate is essential for normal brain function.[84,85] It helps prevent hyperhomocysteinemia, which is associated with increased risk of cardiovascular disease, Parkinson's, Alzheimer's, and other dementia.[86] Green leafy vegetables and asparagus are rich sources of folate and provide the basis for its name. Citrus fruit juices, legumes, and fortified cereals are also excellent sources of folate. It is estimated that 20 percent of Americans have relatively less-effective enzymes for absorbing and using folate, due to a problem with their methylation enzymes (see the Toxicology chapter regarding why you may wish to take methyl folate instead of regular folate).

• How much folate can I safely take each day?
At very high doses (greater than 1,000-2,000 micrograms), folate can trigger the same kinds of nervous system-related symptoms that it is ordinarily used to prevent. These symptoms include insomnia, malaise, irritability, and intestinal dysfunction. Primarily for these reasons, the Institute of Medicine at the National Academy of Sciences set a tolerable UL in 1998 of 1,000 micrograms (mcg) for men and women 19 years and older. This UL was only designed to apply to "synthetic folate," defined as folate obtained from supplements and fortified foods. Taking mega doses of vitamins and nutrients can lead to the body absorbing toxic levels. However, if the kidneys and liver are functioning normally, the body will absorb micronutrients from food without reaching toxic levels. That is another reason to rely on food as the primary source for the micronutrients listed.

Other key micronutrients for mitochondria
There are many other micronutrients, not considered vitamins, which are important for optimal mitochondrial function. I have listed some that have been extensively studied in the laboratory and have been shown to be beneficial for mitochondrial health in studies of animals and humans.

Co-enzyme Q
Co-enzyme Q is an important ingredient in the mitochondrial process to generate ATP and it is a potent intracellular antioxidant. It has been used successfully to reduce the severity of migraines, neuropathies, and dementia.[87-89] Excellent food sources include wheat germ and dark green, leafy vegetables like kale and spinach, and organ meats such as liver, tongue, and heart. Unfortunately, gluten is also present in wheat germ, which means it should be avoided by those who have multiple sclerosis.

Alpha-Lipoic acid
Several studies suggest that treatment with alpha-lipoic acid (ALA) may help reduce pain, burning, itching, tingling, and numbness in people who have nerve damage (called peripheral neuropathy) caused by diabetes.[90-93] ALA acid has been used in Europe for years for this purpose. Good food sources of ALA include spinach, broccoli, beef, yeast (particularly brewer's yeast), and certain organ meats (such as the kidney and heart).

L-carnitine
The chemical structure of the bio-molecule called L-carnitine is related to the B vitamins and assists the mitochondria with utilizing fatty acids as a potential source of energy. L-carnitine also helps in the improvement of muscle strength in neuromuscular-disorder-affected individuals and has been associated with decreased oxidative stress and decreased aging in animal studies.[94-96] L-carnitine and Alpha-lipoic acid have been shown to be a potent combination, providing protection to mitochondria and slowing the effect of aging in animals, but definitive studies have not been completed in humans. The greatest amounts of L-carnitine can be found in dairy products and red meat (eaten raw or very rare is the best way to absorb the nutrient).

Resveratrol
This compound is a polyphpenol (a plant-based compound with antioxi-

dant properties) potent intracellular antioxidant and is found in grapes, red wine, purple grape juice, peanuts, and some berries. It has been associated with decreased aging and neuroprotection in multiple studies.[97-103]

Creatine Monohydrate

Creatine functions to increase the availability of cellular ATP and has been used by weight lifters to help increase their muscle size. Creatine acts by donating a phosphate ion during ATP production to increase the availability of ATP. A couple of studies have shown creatine to be helpful in the brain and muscles of those with neurologically caused weakness and additional studies are underway. Several studies have demonstrated that taking additional creatine has been neuroprotective to a variety of insults and has helped improve and maintain muscle strength in people with Parkinson's and the frail elderly.[104-112] I have used creatine for several years for that reason. The most common risk with taking creatine is an increased risk of kidney stones, particularly if one does not maintain good hydration.

The best food sources of creatine are fish and red meat. Wild game is considered to be the richest source of creatine. The body can also make some creatine in the liver.

Micronutrients for Neurotransmitter Support

A variety of body chemistry imbalances can occur in patients with MS. Excess glutamate in the brain is very common, particularly in the setting of chronic pain. The excessive glutamate can also lead to excito-toxicity, damaging and eventually killing brain cells. There are a number of foods that can be eaten to decrease the toxicity from excessive glutamate. Other neurotransmitters like serotonin and norepinephrine can be influenced by your nutrition as well.

GABA enhancement/glutamate lowering:

Magnesium blocks excessive stimulation from glutamate. It will decrease excito-toxicity when there is too much glutamate in the brain (often seen in patients with MS, chronic pain, anxiety, seizures, and/or mood disorders). Magnesium has been shown to be helpful in reducing the severity of tension headaches and migraines[113-122] and has been shown to be neuroprotective in animal models of brain injury.[123,124] Magnesium is the important center of chlorophyll, much like iron is the center of hemoglobin in our blood. Because people eat so few green leaves, and because stress tends to cause magnesium wasting, many Americans are relatively depleted in their magnesium stores. Good sources include pumpkin seeds, sesame seeds, sunflower seeds, spinach, Swiss chard, black beans, and pinto beans. Several experts have suggested that consuming 500 mg to 800 mg of magnesium per day may help decrease excito-toxicity. The primary side effect from excessive magnesium is diarrhea.

The most common way to take magnesium directly is Milk of Magnesia or MOM, a common over-the-counter treatment for constipation. To avoid the diarrhea side effect, use the tablet form of MOM and gradually increase the number of tablets taken each day until bowel movements are soft. Another effective way to increase magnesium in the body is to absorb it through the skin by taking Epsom Salt baths (magnesium sulfate). It is the magnesium in Epsom Salt that accounts for the soothing effect of taking Epsom Salt baths. It is an excellent way to calm anxiety and lower stress.

Organic Sulfur is needed to generate GABA. Sources include foods from the onion family (garlic, leeks, onion, and chives) and cruciferous family (cabbage, kale, collards, broccoli, cauliflower, radishes, and kohlrabi).

Taurine has been shown to help prevent epileptic seizures[123-127] and to be useful in the prevention of cardiac arrhythmias or heartbeat irregularities, atherosclerosis, and congestive heart failure (in animal studies).[123,124,128-134] Several neurologists and psychiatrists have suggested some of their patients use one to two grams a day in divided doses to support the generation of GABA as a strategy to protect the brain or to assist in the treatment of mood disorders.[123,124,135-138] Fish and shellfish are good sources of taurine.

Glutathione is very important to the generation of GABA. It is manufactured inside the cell, from its precursor amino acids: glycine, glutamate, and cysteine. Hence, food sources or supplements taken to increase glutathione must either provide the precursors of glutathione or enhance its production by some other means. The manufacture of glutathione in cells is primarily limited by the levels of cysteine, a precursor amino acid containing sulfur.

Strategies to Increase Glutathione:

N-acetylcysteine (NAC) is considered the most cost-effective strategy to increase intracellular glutathione.[124,136,137] It is a key component to the generation of GABA. The recommended daily allowance for a 150-pound adult is two grams a day. It is found in a variety of foods, including poultry, yogurt, egg yolks, red peppers, garlic, onions, broccoli, Brussels sprouts, and other cruciferous vegetables. It is also found in oats, wheat germ, asparagus, and avocado. *N-acetyl cysteine* has proven, in numerous scientific studies and clinical trials, to boost intracellular production of glutathione. It has been approved by the FDA for several types of treatments.

Because it is an effective helper in the detoxification process, NAC (as the brand name Mucomyst) is approved by the FDA for treatment of acetaminophen overdose and to help protect the kidneys from the toxic effects of IV contrast used in some x-ray studies. Because of glutathione's tremendous importance in keeping the mitochondria healthy in the lungs, kidneys, and brain, NAC is commonly used in the treatment of lung diseases like cystic fibrosis, bronchitis, and asthma. Several neurologists and psychiatrists have asked patients to use one to two grams of NAC each day to support GABA generation in the brain. For some individuals, however, diarrhea occurs at doses more than 500 mg per day.

Milk thistle is a powerful antioxidant and supports the brain, liver, and kidneys in animal studies by preventing the depletion of glutathione.[139-147] Silymarin is the active compound of milk thistle. Because it has been shown to help prevent depletion of glutathione, it is considered helpful to the detoxification process in the liver. It is also thought to protect the liver from toxins, such as carbon tetrachloride and alcohol. You can also get milk thistle seeds from health food stores, which can be ground in your coffee grinder and added to tea or smoothies (1/4 to 1 teaspoon) to help support your mitochondria.

Turmeric is used in the treatment of brain cells, called *astrocytes*. The Indian curry spice curcumin (turmeric) has been found to increase expression of the enzymes that are important to the manufacturing of GABA (glutathione S-transferase), leading to the protection of neurons exposed to oxidant stress.[148-151] Using turmeric regularly in your cooking, or in teas and smoothies, can help support your brain's ability to make GABA.

Selenium is a co-factor for the enzyme *glutathione peroxidase*, which helps generate glutathione in the mitochondria.[152,153] As such, it has also been shown to be neuroprotective.[152,154,155] Good sources include fish, mushrooms, tofu, free-range chicken, turkey, and venison. Too much selenium can cause toxic effects, including gastrointestinal upset, brittle nails, hair loss, and mild nerve damage. But that is extremely unlikely if you are using food sources and taking only what is found in a multi-vitamin/mineral combination. Deriving selenium from food sources has not been associated with any toxic effects.

Norepinephrine lowering substances:

Theanine has been shown to be neuroprotective in animal studies,[156,157] as well as improving cognition and concentration and reducing anxiety and depression.[158-160] It has a favorable impact on the production of several important neurotransmitters that regulate mood and attention.[161-165] Theanine is an amino acid found uniquely in green tea, particularly in Matcha tea, used in the Japanese Buddhist monasteries and as part of the tea ceremony for centuries. Matcha tea is brilliant emerald green and has more antioxidants and theanine than the green tea brewed with dried tea leaves. Several cups a day are beneficial to help lower brain norepinephrine, decrease distractibility, and improve concentration. Doses commonly used range from 300 mg to 500 mg per day.

Serotonin enhancement:

<u>Aerobic exercise</u>: Physical activity boosts the brain serotonin levels.[166,167] Thirty minutes of activity will elevate one's serotonin. Even a brisk walk is helpful for the body and mind.

<u>Vitamin D</u>: Many adolescents, adults, and elderly individuals are vitamin D deficient.[168-171] In addition to being important in bone development, vitamin D provides important support to immune function, lowers the risk of autoimmune diseases,[172-177] lowers the risk of cancer,[178-181] and is important in maintaining normal mood.[182-184] Many physicians advise patients to routinely take 2000 international units (IU) of vitamin D each day. Doses higher than 2000 IU should be monitored by a physician. If someone is low in vitamin D, physicians often use either vitamin D2 at 50,000 IU weekly, or vitamin D3 at 8,000 to 10,000 IU daily. The vitamin D level is checked every three months until the total level is midrange to slightly above midrange. Often doses of 4000 IU daily are required for people to maintain their vitamin D levels in the midrange. The hazard of excessive vitamin D levels is too much calcium in the blood stream, which can cause kidney stones, confusion, and seizures. It is best to have your physician follow your vitamin D level to make sure that your vitamin D level is in the upper half of the range.

<u>St. John's Wort</u> is an herb that has been used to treat mood disorders. Studies have shown it to be comparable to placebo in treating depression. Notably, multiple studies have also demonstrated that St. Johnswort has the same effectiveness as the family of antidepressant medicines that include Prozac (selective serotonin reuptake inhibitors, or SSRIs).[185-187] Be-

cause St. Johnswort affects how your body metabolizes some medicines, it is very important to tell your physicians and your pharmacist if you are taking it to avoid dangerous drug interactions.

Minerals

<u>Iodine</u> is important to brain health because it is involved in making myelin. It is also important to the mitochondrial processes involved in removing toxic heavy metals. Additionally, iodine is important in the manufacture of many hormones and the controlled killing of bacteria. Low iodine levels are associated with mental retardation, thyroid disease, and increased risk of infertility, breast cancer, and prostate cancer. Good sources of iodine include seaweed (especially dried kelp), shellfish, and other seafood.

<u>Zinc</u> is another mineral important to brain health. Low levels of zinc are associated with abnormal taste, depressed immunity, and increased risk of depression. Good sources include seaweed, liver, pumpkin seeds, nutritional yeast, and greens.

<u>Other trace minerals</u> that are important to human health are boron, cobalt, copper, chromium, fluorine, iron, manganese, molybdenum, nickel, silicon, and vanadium. People who have reduced their dietary salt, and do not eat much fish or seaweed, may be short on their trace minerals. Good sources include seaweed, shellfish, iodized sea salt, and nutritional or brewer's yeast. Another way to get trace minerals are soaks in mineral baths, which are a combination of sea salt and magnesium salts.

In summary, micronutrients have important roles to play in brain health and immune function. The standard Western diet is often deficient in multiple vitamins and minerals. Improving the micronutrient content of the diet by increasing the intake of non-starchy vegetables, fruits, nuts, seeds, fish, shellfish, and organ meats is very important to maintaining healthy function of the mitochondria, normal immune function, protection against cancer, and normal brain function. Eat more greens and colorful fruits and vegetables, meat and fish rich in omega-3 fats, and ensure you get plenty of minerals by eating more seaweed, nutritional yeast, and shellfish. Food is a superior way to obtain these nutrients, although some individuals may require both a diet rich in healthy foods as well as supplementation of specific key nutrients. Discuss any supplements that you are considering taking with your doctor or pharmacist to be sure there will be no unexpected adverse interactions with your other medicines or health issues. It is possible to inadvertently take excessive levels of a nutrient when using supplements. This is why it is crucial that you alert your pharmacists and medical providers if you are using or considering using supplements.

Chapter Five
NEUROPROTECTION

Neuroprotection is the means by which the brain and nervous system protects itself against deterioration. While the public is hoping stem cell research will provide the cure for MS and other brain disorders, such treatments are likely decades away. All of us, however, produce stem cells in our brains now if we are producing brain growth factors. These special hormones, or *nerve growth factors*, are made in the brain. These growth factors are associated with increasing the growth of axons, dendrites, and myelin within the brain and spinal cord. Our brains are continuously pruning the unused connections (dendrites and axons) in our brains. If we have enough brain growth factors and are learning new physical or mental skills, our brains generate nerve growth factors. These factors signal the brain cells to begin making nerve sprouts, which will grow into new dendrites and axons. The good news is that there are a number of things you can do to boost the amount of nerve growth factors your brain makes each day.

A higher amount of nerve growth factors are also associated with greater levels of repair activities in the brain. The level is decreased in the persons who have MS. However, several studies have demonstrated that these growth factors can be increased, even in the MS patients. The protection of brain cells appears to be most promising with sodium channel blockers (such as amitryptiline, the lidocaine family of drugs, and lithium). Although the data in human studies is early, the following techniques and supplements have been shown to be associated with increased levels of either brain-derived neurotrophic factor or nerve growth factor. They have been demonstrated to offer protection against a wide variety of situations harmful to the brain, such as inadequate oxygen and toxic chemicals used in the animal studies to create neurological disorders. Also, other nutrients such as omega-3 fats, especially docosohexanoic acid (DHA), resveratrol, and sulfur, have been shown to boost the production of nerve growth factors.

Thirty minutes of aerobic exercise has been shown to increase a number of the nerve growth factors, which promote the generation of new nerve cells, connectivity between the cells, and myelin repair (very important in MS).[188] This has been helpful in other neurodegenerative disorders, such as Parkinson's, Alzheimer's, and MS. Exercise has also been helpful in reducing depression and anxiety.

Thirty minutes of brain exercise in the form of solving puzzles (e.g., sudoku or crossword), learning new cognitive skills (e.g., adult education classes, new computer programs), or new physical skills (e.g., juggling) has been shown to increase a number of the nerve-growth factors,[189-191] which promote the generation of new nerve cells. Nintendo's Brain Age is an example of a method for mental training. This has also been helpful in the treatment of neurodegenerative disorders and psychiatric disorders.

Gingko is available as an herbal supplement over the counter and has been shown to be helpful in slowing the progress of dementia.[192]

Co-Enzyme Q is a mitochondrial nutrient. It has been shown in several studies to slow the progression of Parkinson's and Alzheimer's.[193-196] If you use co-enzyme Q, discuss it with your pharmacist to be sure there are no interactions with your other medicines. It has been associated with increasing the potency of certain thyroid medications and causing palpitations. Excellent sources of co-enzyme Q include organ meat, green leafy vegetables, nutritional yeast, wheat germ organ meat, nuts, and seeds. However, since wheat germ also includes gluten, those who are avoiding gluten should also avoid wheat germ.

Lithium, in prescription drug form as lithium carbonate, is used primarily to treat bipolar disorder, also known as manic-depressive disorder. The drug is effective in treating the mania in particular. It has been shown to be helpful in protecting the brain against atrophy of the hippocampus, which is often seen in bipolar disorder and is a potent stimulater of brain derived growth factors (hormones secreted in the brain to stimulate growth of brain cells).[149,197-199] It has also been shown to slow and reverse the damage done in the animal model used to study multiple sclerosis.[200] Because lithium interferes with the kidneys' ability to concentrate urine, it is important to drink plenty of fluids when taking lithium.

Lithium is being studied as a treatment intervention in several neurodegenerative disorders. It has been helpful for some, but not all. Those with neurodegenerative diseases may wish to discuss with their physicians and pharmacists whether lithium's ability to stimulate the brain growth factors may be beneficial to them. However, be aware that lithium has the potential for adverse drug interactions. That is why it is important that your physicians and pharmacists be aware of the entire list of drugs, vitamins and supplements which you take.

<u>Sleep</u> is an important anti-inflammation process for the body. In my clinical practice I see many people with traumatic brain injury and post-traumatic stress disorder that have disrupted sleep. Helping them achieve a more normal sleep pattern without relying on drug medications is very helpful. There are two hormones that I work to correct is those circumstances. These are cortisol (the stress hormone) and melatonin (the sleep hormone).

Cortisol is a hormone secreted in response to stress and helps the body be prepared to flee from danger or fight the impending danger. That is why it is also known as "flight or fight." Melatonin is secreted by the brain in response to darkness. It is associated with the induction and maintenance of sleep. However, when the cortisol is chronically high, the body stays in a state of constant activation and vigilance. It becomes very difficult to sleep. One of the consequences of chronic activation is high levels of inflammation in the body. Brain cells are stressed and experience early death. Sleep is also diminished.

Because we now have artificial lights, the natural wake-sleep cycle has been disrupted. For many, the use of artificial light lowers the brain's ability to generate melatonin. The consequence is difficulty initiating and maintaining sleep.

In my practice, I ask people to lower their stress hormones and boost their sleep hormones. Stress hormones can be lowered by quiet time, meditation, guided imagery, prayer, time in nature, and taking a soak in a magnesium salts (Epsom salts) bath. Other strategies can include the use of digitally reengineered music to induce relaxation. One example of such products is an audio CD titled *Zen Meditate* by iMusic. Another company, the EOC Institute, has three audio CDs, *Enlightenment, Ascension,* and *Balance*, which have also been engineered to generate alpha, beta, and theta brain waves that lead to meditative levels of relaxation and health benefits.

In addition, I have suggested my patients take 1 mg of melatonin an hour before they wish to go to sleep. Melatonin is available over the counter in the supplement section of most pharmacies and has relatively few side effects. Certainly, fewer side effects than another over-the-counter substance, diphenhydramine, which is associated with impaired balance, coordination, and judgment, especially in those who are elderly or in poor health.

In summary, there are a number of strategies one can use to help protect brain cells. Physical activity and mental training in the form of lifelong learning stimulates the release of important growth factors and neurotrophins for the brain. Improving the quality of sleep through the reduction of stress hormones is important also and taking melatonin is helpful. Supplements and medications that have shown promise in some animal model studies include co-enzyme Q and lithium.

Chapter Six
WHY FOOD MATTERS IN MS

There are three main ways food can make trouble for individuals, especially those with MS: toxins from the use of herbicides and pesticides, deficient micronutrient intake, and food allergies and sensitization.

Toxins are present in any food that is grown with the help of pesticides and insecticides. The best options to deal with this are to grow your own food or buy local organic food when you can. Wash all produce carefully, especially if you buy non-organic. The more fragile the food (e.g., raspberries) the less likely you can remove the pesticides from the food through washing. Some produce, such as lettuce, berries, and celery, have high amounts of pesticide residue, so get those organically if you can. You need healthy mitochondria to excrete those toxins. If you do not have healthy mitochondria, then you will steadily accumulate more toxins in fat cells and your brain as a result.

Micronutrients and the deficiency of the Standard American Diet (SAD) have been discussed previously.

Insulin is a hormone produced by the pancreas, which is vital to the body in some amounts and inflammatory in higher amounts.[201-203] Insulin controls the levels of blood sugar (glucose). The more insulin our bodies need to make to control our blood sugar, the more inflammation molecules we make as well. A diet that does not generate rapid climbs in blood sugar does not require as much insulin. The best diet to lower the insulin levels focuses on non-starchy vegetables, protein sources, and whole fruit, and avoids or minimizes grains. Whole grains are absorbed more slowly and therefore generate less insulin. Simple sugars and starches, such as those found in corn syrup, candy, sugared drinks, juice without pulp, white potatoes, pastries, pastas, and white bread make our blood sugar rise rapidly and should be avoided.

Food allergies and sensitivities are also a contributor. Celiac disease, for example, causes the body to make antibodies against gluten (found in wheat, rye, and barley).[204-206] The symptoms are not just contained in the belly and gut. People with celiac disease can also have skin problems, joint problems, fatigue, personality changes, mood problems, weakness, and pain. Some patients have come to their physicians with severe neurological problems and severe changes on their brain MRIs and, as a result, have been diagnosed with multiple sclerosis. But it is important to consider the possibility of gluten sensitivity; there are multiple case reports in the literature of patients who have had confirmed neurological or psychological disorders who were found to have gluten sensitivity as the primary reason for their illnesses.[207-217] After faithfully following a gluten-free diet, their psychological and neurological problems, including abnormal brain scans, resolved over the subsequent year. Anyone who has been diagnosed with MS would benefit from eating a very stringent gluten-free diet for at least a month to help determine what role gluten sensitivity may have in their disease.

If we can have that level of damage to the brain as a result of sensitivity to gluten, it is logical to consider that sensitivity to other foods might generate similar levels of damage to the body and brain. Anyone with MS whose symptoms are still bothersome would benefit from considering the possibility of food sensitivities as a factor that is keeping their disease active.

This is a complex issue to resolve, because people can end up sensitized to many different food items. We know that seventy percent of those with gluten sensitivity have their symptoms completely resolved with gluten avoidance. The other thirty percent have additional food sensitivities that must be identified and eliminated in order to improve symptoms.

So how do we figure out who is sensitive to what foods? For several reasons, it is not easy to determine. Blood tests can identify some of the sensitivities, but not all, and, although most reactions occur quickly, some reactions to food occur up to seventy-two hours after ingestion. As a result, the most effective way to confirm food sensitivities is through an elimination diet, using a food diary and symptom diary for a minimum of one month.

There are many books devoted to celiac disease and gluten-free diets. The Internet provides many sources of additional information.

Two approaches to identifying food sensitivities

1. <u>Gradual food reintroduction</u> is the most stringent application of a food diet. This method asks the individual to eat only the most non-sensitizing foods available for a week, and then gradually reintroduce one food item per week. The individual keeps a symptom record. If no symptoms of any type occur in that week, the food item is identified as safe and added to the list of allowed foods. Over several months, food items are gradually returned to the diet. Because of this slow, careful process, it is possible to identify with precision what foods cause which symptoms, and eliminate that particular food from the diet. But many people are not willing or capable of carrying out that kind of protocol.

2. <u>Elimination diets</u> are a more moderate approach. Elimination diets require a lot of advance planning for them to work. The person with MS is advised to initially eliminate the most common sources of food allergy from their diet. This includes wheat, eggs, milk, and legumes (including peanuts, soy and cashews). They are given a chart that lays out a four-day rotation plan with menu suggestions. The goal is for the individual to eat from different food families every day so that no one food is eaten more frequently than every four days. The individual must keep a food and symptom diary.

Because almost all food-allergy symptoms occur within seventy-two hours, in the event of possible symptoms, a food diary is essential to know which of the food items eaten in the prior three days were previously identified as safe in the past and which foods were newly introduced in that time period. The possible culprit is then eliminated from the diet.

If desired, the eliminated food could be tried again in four to six months. Some people have a few severe food allergies and others which are milder. If the food that causes a mild allergic reaction is eliminated for six months, the lining of the gut heals. Then if the gut encounters that food only on occasion, the cells may tolerate it without causing a major antibody response. The other benefit of an elimination diet is that it increases the variety of our food intake, often improving micronutrient content in the long run.

Eating out at restaurants and eating processed foods is challenging for people using an elimination diet or the gradual food reintroduction method to identify food allergies and sensitivities. You must read labels carefully, and be willing to ask the waiter about what foods may be included in the dish you are ordering. The simplest approach is to avoid eating processed food and eating out, particularly while you are first going through the process.

There are many books available on the issue of food sensitivities and micronutrients to help with designing menus that can work for you. These include the following books and their associated Web sites:

- *The Whole Life Nutrition Cookbook*: http://www.wholelifenutrition.net/
- *The World's Healthiest Foods*: http://www.whfoods.com/
- *The MS Recovery Diet*: http://msrecoverydiet.com/
- Information about obtaining a healthy group of bacteria in your colon can be found at: http://www.amazon.com/Restoring-Your-Digestive-Health-Transfom/dp/07582028220

Gluten-free diet resources:
- www.celiac.com and http://www.breadsfromanna.com/recipes (Anna Sobaski is an Iowa City chef who has gluten-free mixes you can make at home. Our family has used them quite successfully!)
- Vegan resources: http://www.vegan-food.net/ (No animal protein; site helps you find substitutions for eggs, cheese, and dairy products, in addition to being meat-free.)
- Asthon Embry has written extensively on connections between diet and MS: http://www.direct-ms.org/bestbet.html

Gut Health and Bacteria
In addition to the problem of food allergies, people can have problems with the wrong bacteria in their gut. The typical person has one trillion cells in their bodies and 100 trillion bacteria in their bowels, their nose and lungs, and genital tract. Over hundreds of generations we co-evolved with our bacteria. The bacteria take the food we eat and digest it, making byproducts that are used by other bacteria. As a species, we have learned how to use all those byproducts in our own bodies, such as the vitamin K made by the bacteria in our gut, or we have created enzymes that safely dispose of

the byproducts we can't use. The result is that we and gut bacteria thrive together.

Now that we have shifted our ancient diets into a diet that emphasizes sugar, white flour, and dairy, new and different bacteria and parasites grow in our bowels. They make new byproducts, many of which our species has not seen before. The result is that our bowels now grow pseudomonas, clostridium difficile, streptococcus, and staphylococcus and proteus species. Toxins are produced that worsen inflammation and make the symptoms of depression, arthritis, and diabetes much harder to control.[218-225] Using probiotics to reintroduce familiar bacteria to our gut is helpful. But if we don't stop eating the sugar, white flour, and white potatoes, the harmful bacteria will continue to outnumber the helpful bacteria. We will continue to not be well.

It is important, therefore, to change our diets back to eating what our ancestors would have eaten thousands of years ago. That means eating greens, colors, and high-quality protein. It means stopping the sugar, stopping the white flour, stopping the dairy and the gluten grains. Probiotics are helpful. But you still need to change the diet back to what our species ate for generations to maintain healthy bowel bacteria. Then you have less inflammation and greater health and vitality.[226]

Summary

Food matters, especially to people with diseases such as MS. If you can, grow some of your own food (organically). Buy organic foods whenever possible. Try eliminating the most common allergen offenders — gluten, eggs, milk, and peanuts. Keep a food/symptom diary. Try an elimination diet with a four-day food rotation and consult with a nutritionist or other healthcare provider familiar with elimination diets. Exercise can help increase the brain growth factors and speed healing, but without the needed micronutrients and lower levels of inflammation, you won't get far. The quality of the food you eat is important, but equally important is the avoidance of foods to which you are sensitive. For some individuals, finding a Functional Medicine healthcare practitioner that is familiar with elimination diets and food sensitivity can be very helpful.

Chapter Seven
THE POISONS IN OUR FOOD, WATER, AND AIR

Rachel Carson, in *Silent Spring*, published in 1962, wrote:

> For the first time in the history of the world, every human being is now subjected to contact with dangerous chemicals, from the moment of conception until death. In the less than two decades of their use, the synthetic pesticides have been so thoroughly distributed throughout the animate and inanimate world that they occur virtually everywhere.[227]

What do we know now, nearly fifty years later, about the impact of these compounds on health and the health of our children? In this chapter I'll focus on how these new chemicals are impacting our health, and what we can do about our toxic load in addition to choosing organically grown foods.

Since World War II, we have had to revolutionize the way work was performed, the way food was grown and prepared for consumption, and how our living environments were maintained. Instead of relying on human labor, we increasingly used newly created chemicals to fertilize the soil, kill weeds and insects, eliminate stains, odors, and germs, keep food from spoiling, and more. The list of ways in which chemicals now interface with all of our lives is very long. These modern chemicals saved hours and hours of human labor and allowed for rapid increases in the production of food at lower costs per unit. Most of the small family farms of our grand-parents and great-grandparents have been replaced by larger and larger farms, requiring ever larger equipment and more chemical applications and innovations, until finally, some genetically modified soybean and corn seeds can now produce their own pesticides in the plants, courtesy of pesticide-producing genes inserted into their DNA.

The term for new compounds that interact with biological systems is *xenobiotics*. These compounds interact with the cells, receptors, and mito-chondria in ways that may interfere with the normal function of cells. When that happens, a change occurs. When it is helpful, the compound is often marketed as a medicine. When it is harmful, the compound is regulated as a toxin and a level is chosen to identify when the food, water, or air is safe for human consumption. The tests are expensive to conduct and are gen-erally done one compound at a time and on laboratory animals. However, we don't interact with one compound at a time. We interact with all of the hundreds, if not thousands, of chemical compounds that have made their way into our food, water, and indoor and outdoor environments.

In addition to the chemicals in the food supply, there are the chemicals in the world in which we live. For example, wood is treated with arsenic to keep it from rotting. Arsenic-treated wood, banned from structures in zoos because it is too toxic, is often used for human play structures. Chil-dren who play on treated wooden structures consume arsenic at levels ten times the amount allowable in water or food by the EPA, because children commonly touch their hands to their mouths.[228-231] Furthermore, studies that examined chemicals in the cord blood of babies at birth and in human breast milk have documented the presence of pesticides, flame retardants, plastics, mercury, lead, arsenic, and numerous pesticides, many of which had been banned for years.[232-236] Mercury, lead, and aluminum are heavy metals that poison many key enzymes in the body. They are present in the food chain, the water supply, and the air.

Coal mining and burning coal for electricity deposits millions of tons of lead and mercury into the air each year.[237] And elevated heavy metal con-tamination is associated with a much higher rate of early onset dementia, and higher rates of autism, learning disabilities, bipolar disorder, refractory depression, and other neuropsychiatric diseases.[238,239] Another major source of mercury is dental amalgam, also known as silver fillings.[240] The amount of mercury in the mouth is associated with the amount of mercury in the brain.[241] If one's body happens to have enzymes that are less effective at metabolizing and excreting the mercury, then the amount of mercury given off as vapors from the dental amalgam is more likely to be absorbed into the brain. Gradually, neurobehavioral problems can accumulate, which are difficult to diagnose and difficult to treat.

Endocrine disrupters, or EDs, are compounds that affect the hormonal signaling in our bodies. Hormones are the molecules used by our bodies to regulate our sex traits (estrogen and testosterone), our metabolism (thyroid hormones), our energy (cortisol, epinephrine, and norepinephrine) and our size (growth hormone). These can be found in detergents, fragrances, cosmetics, sun screens, and pesticides, as well as the hormones injected in animals raised for meat production. The EDs can affect estrogen, testosterone, thyroid, and cortisol receptors — and thereby affect our health, metabolism, and our energy reserves. They are blamed, in part, for the falling fertility in females, a 40% drop in sperm counts worldwide, and are thought to contribute to the earlier onset of puberty.[242-245]

Heavy metals and pesticide exposures have been associated with multiple brain-related health problems. Mercury, for example, is a known neurotoxin.[246-250] However, researchers have not found a strong association between dental mercury or mercury in vaccines and MS in multiple epidemiologic studies.[251-256] Yet studies have shown that the burden of mercury in the brain is associated with the amount of dental amalgam in the mouth.[257] Part of the reason for this discrepancy could be related to *single nucleotide polymorphisms* (also called SNPs) of the DNA that provide the instructions for making the methylation and sulfation enzymes our cells use to remove toxins from the body in the process called detoxification. People who have been shown to have these SNPs have less efficient enzymes for removing toxins, have been associated with increased susceptibility to arsenic and other heavy metals,[258-260] and are more likely to have mental health problems or neurological problems. It is therefore not surprising that multiple authors have found associations between early onset Parkinson's disease, heavy metal and/or pesticide exposures, and these SNPs.[260-266] Thus, it is possible that the individuals with multiple sclerosis or with Parkinson's disease have enzymes that are less effective at removing toxins and are therefore much more sensitive to the various toxins in the environment. People with such SNPs have a much higher requirement for B vitamins or other mitochondrial nutrients and an increased risk of developing neurotoxicity and chronic diseases involving the brain, heart, and joints.[267-280]

As stated earlier, we are exposed to hundreds, if not thousands, of chemicals simultaneously. Because of our own unique biochemical individuality, courtesy of our DNA, how those toxins will affect the biochemistry in our cells will vary from individual to individual. Our mitochondria must manage the chemical reactions that are necessary for the body to transform the foreign or xenobiotic chemicals into forms we can excrete in our bile, sweat, or urine. Mitochondria that have all of the nutrients they need for optimal function can more easily add the necessary sulfur and methyl groups in order for our bodies to excrete these toxic compounds. In that case, the damage done to our tissues by toxins is relatively minimal, because we are able to excrete all the toxins that are absorbed each day. Our total toxic load then remains zero (i.e., toxic load equals our toxins absorbed minus the toxins excreted) and we remain healthy.

On the other hand, if our diet is poor, our mitochondria do not have enough B vitamins, coenzyme Q, and antioxidants to use. When we cannot get rid of all the toxins each day, we begin to store toxins in the fat tissues. That results in toxins being stored in the fat deposits in our bodies, including the brain, which has a large amount of fat in the myelin. If toxins accumulate, many enzymes, including many involved in detoxification, are poisoned by the toxins, making removal of the toxins even more difficult. Toxin levels rise further, leading to greater levels of oxidative stress and other damage to the cells. As the cells become damaged, more inflammation cytokines are generated. The elevated cytokines drive the production of more inflammation-related molecules, which, in turn, makes more cytokines. Eventually the body will begin to make antibodies against itself. As the auto-antibodies circulate, they will call upon the immune cells to attack the body.

If you want to excrete more toxins, you need to have healthy mitochondria, because your mitochondria do the work of metabolizing the toxins. Therefore, you will want to maximize your intake of B vitamins, coenzyme Q, and antioxidants. The specific enzymes that transform synthetic chemicals so they can be excreted in the urine, bile, or sweat involve the addition of methyl groups or a sulfur group. These enzymes are called phase I and phase II enzymes. Foods that support these enzymes include cruciferous vegetables, allicin (garlic and onion vegetables), and brightly colored fruits and vegetables — exactly the foods I stress in the Wahls Diet. At the end of the book, you will find several figures that list the nutrients and foods that support the detoxification pathways in the liver, kidney and sweat glands. In the recipes chapter you will find recipes for making your own "detox smoothies" and "detox teas." As always, be sure to discuss with your doctor before beginning to use them on a regular basis.

Since your toxic load is equal to the toxins you absorb each day minus the toxins you excrete each day, there are two prongs to reducing your toxic load. First, you can reduce your exposure; second, you can work to improve your body's ability to excrete the toxins you absorb. We absorb toxins through our digestive system, our skin, and our lungs. If you want to minimize exposure then you need to reduce your potential sources of contact through food, water, and air. The obvious place to start is with the food we eat. Consider shifting to organic foods and growing what you can yourself, whether it is a small pot of herbs in your window or a large garden plot. For the food you buy, look for the USDA label certifying the food was grown using organic methods. You can also check a number of Internet sites for information on organic foods. A great international organization promoting the return to the eating of good clean foods is Slow Foods. More information about them can be found at **http://www.slowfoodusa.org/**.

Other sources of toxins include the water we drink and use to bathe and swim. Reverse osmosis water filters reduce the risk of water-borne toxins and are available commercially. The halogens added to preserve food (bromine), water (chlorine), and to lower risk of dental cavities (fluoride), all increase the dietary requirement of iodine, a necessary nutrient to make myelin and important for the detoxification of heavy metals.

Because air pollution is increasingly a factor in many environments, you may also want to consider how to reduce the air pollution in your home and work environment as well. Reduce your use of indoor chemicals; use more natural cleaning products, stop the monthly visit from pest control services, and avoid dry cleaning your clothes (at least air them out considerably). You may also wish to consider buying an air filtration system if air quality is known to be poor in your locale. Live green plants can help improve air quality. More information can be found at: **http://www.wolvertonenviron-mental.com/airFAQ.htm**.

An excellent resource to learn more about how to support the mitochondria's ability to detoxify are books by Dr. Mark Hyman. He has several references for the public. These include: *Detox in a Box, The Five Forces of Wellness: The Ultra Prevention System for Living an Active, Age-Defying, Disease-Free Life* and *The Ultra Mind Solution*: *Fix Your Broken Brain by Healing Your Broken Body.* More information can be found at his Web site: **http://www.drhyman.com/**. Dr. Hyman discusses the benefits and hazards of additional strategies, such as increasing excretion through sauna use (sweating), binding toxins through the use of clay baths to pulls toxins out through the skin, and binding toxins through intravenous medication so they can be more easily excreted in the urine and/or bile.

Two years after intensive nutrition to support my mitochondria, I completed a toxicology screen on myself. The results were sobering. I had modest elevations of mercury, which is not surprising since I have several amalgam fillings. I had normal levels of fluoride, but marked elevations of bromide. My iodine stores were low, even though I had been taking supplemental iodine for three months. I had elevations of barium, aluminum, cadmium, cesium, gadolinium, nickel, platinum, rubidium, thallium, tungsten, and uranium. The likely sources for the gadolinium are the multiple MRI examinations. The others heavy metals, others than aluminum, were probably ground water contamination from growing up on an Iowa farm and living in communities that used treated river water for municipal water. No doubt, my heavy metal burden was higher two years ago than it is now.

So what have I done to boost my own detoxification now that I have gotten that toxicology report back to reduce my toxic load? First, I have since added more algae (rotating between different algaes — Klamath blue green, spirulina, and chlorella) to my morning smoothies, since they all bind heavy metals in the gut. That way I don't recycle the heavy metals excreted into the bile back into my blood stream. Second, I take a clay foot bath every morning, along with a twenty minute sauna. Third, in the middle of the night, when I go to the bathroom, I take an edible clay tablet by mouth along with a couple of fiber tablets. To further reduce toxins absorbed, I put in a reverse-osmosis water filter in my home. I am much more careful about eating organic. My physician also advised that I take one teaspoon of algae once or twice a day, and eat seaweed several times a week or take a teaspoon of dried kelp daily for the trace minerals and iodine. In addition, I was advised to add, at minimum, 500 mg of niacinamide and 200 mg of riboflavin daily

Let me explain how clay pulls toxins out of the body. The molecules of clay are positively charged and heavy metals are typically negatively charged. As a result, the clay will pull the metal ions out through the skin, if you are taking a clay foot bath or whole bath. Alternatively, one can take edible clay tablets by mouth, since the lining of our small bowel is the equivalent of a football field in size. However, the clay, in addition to absorbing heavy metals, pesticides, and other toxins, will also absorb medications from your blood stream. Therefore, if you are taking medications and plan to use clay baths to support detoxification, you must be mindful that the clay will also remove the medications you take from your blood stream, right along with the toxins. You will need to time the clay baths and/or edible clay tablets at the nadir (ideally, just before you would be taking the medication), so that while your body is absorbing the medicines, your clay is not also busy removing the medication from your system

After adding those things, within just one month I experienced another boost in energy. I do plan to repeat the heavy metals, bromide, and iodine assessments in 12 months to see where my toxin load is at that time and will continue to follow my toxin levels until they are normalized.

For those who want more information on iodine, iodine and toxin assessments can be found at the Iodine 4 Health Web site: **http://iodine4health. com/**. Additional information on detoxification can be found at a radiation detox site run by Bill Bodri. Although most of us are not radioactive, the information he provides is well cited. He utilizes many publications from experiences with the successful detoxification of the radiation exposures from Hiroshima and Chernobyl. The free e-Book is located at **http://www. radiationdetox.com/**. He provides a long list of specific suggestions of foods to eat that can maximize production of the detoxifying enzymes and provide greater support to the mitochondria as they work to excrete toxins. Like me, he stresses cruciferous and allicin vegetables. He also stresses the benefits of algae and kelp by mouth and the use of clay baths to help pull the toxins through the skin and out of the body.

In summary, toxins are present in our food, water, air, and surrounding environment. Toxic load is the amount of toxins absorbed each day minus the amount of toxins excreted each day. Eating organically grown food is helpful, as is reducing the use of indoor chemicals. Mitochondria add methyl and sulfur groups to toxins so that they can be excreted in the urine, sweat, and bile. Therefore, increasing the intake of vitamins, sulfur, minerals, antioxidants, and phase I and phase II enzyme inducers help the mitochondria excrete toxins. Eating more greens, colored fruits and vegetables, algae, and seaweed is very helpful for supporting the mitochondria's work in detoxification. Increasing the amount of urine, bowel movements, and sweat also increases the excretion of toxins. Using toxin binders like algae, green tea, and clay, either on the skin or orally, can also be helpful.

Chapter Eight
RECIPES

These are a few of my favorite recipes. They provide an excellent source of nutrients that are vital to mitochondria and brain health, and none of the recipes contain gluten, dairy, or eggs. In my case, I focused on adding foods from the cabbage family, onion family, and mushroom family to my diet. I worked to ensure that I had four cups each day from those three food families. Notably, because the cruciferous vegetables will also weakly compete with the iodine receptors, people who eat a lot of cruciferous vegetables should probably modestly increase their intake of iodine and iodide. The best way to do that is to eat more shellfish and sea vegetables.

In a typical day, I will eat 6 cups (600 grams) of collards, kale, or other green leafy vegetables. I will also usually eat 100 grams in each of the three color groups: blue-black, red, and yellow-orange, for a total of 300 grams of antioxidant-rich food. I take one to two tablespoons of nutritional yeast, one to two teaspoons of dried kelp, and a teaspoon of algae in my smoothies each day. I am careful to eat grass-fed meat, free-range chickens, and wild fish to ensure that I have plenty of omega-3 fatty acids. I can feel the difference to my health, general well-being, and MS symptoms within one or two days if I am not able to eat the foods I prefer.

Taking the equivalent amount of micronutrients in pill form would require many hundreds of capsules. Although supplements may be helpful for some people, they play a much smaller role in a person's overall nutrition. You can't expect to take a number of supplements, eat the standard American diet, rich in white flour, white potatoes, sugar and high fructose corn syrup and enjoy good health. Every calorie that is spent, eating white flour (even non-gluten grains), white sugar or high fructose corn syrup that one eats is a calorie spent on starvation. That is because these foods have so few vitamins, minerals, essential fats or other important phytonutrients that your cells will still be starved for important micronutrients. When we become less than healthy, we need all of our calories to be packed with micronutrients. That is why I stress to my patients, white flour, white sugar, high fructose corn syrups are all calories pushing them into worsening disease and micronutrient starvation.

Key to Recipes

Symbol
© Recipe courtesy and copyright the Institute for Functional Medicine

Recipes rich in:
* Omega-3 Fatty Acids
† Sulfur
‡ Anti-Oxidants
§ Bone and Joint Nutrients

Gluten-free, dairy-free, egg-free living
This is difficult to do for many people, particularly at first. All of the recipes included here are free of gluten, dairy, and eggs. I suggest to my patients that they carefully eliminate gluten, dairy, and eggs from their diets for a couple of weeks, and then give themselves a test meal of gluten grains and see how they feel the next three days. If they have no symptoms, then gluten may not be a problem. The following week they should have a dairy test meal, and the week after that an egg test meal. Then they will know if these foods cause them problems.

I've added a couple of recipes that I've made to make gluten-free, dairy-free, and egg-free pancakes, flatbread, and pie. Good resources for additional gluten-free flour mixes for home cooking can be found at http://www.breadsfromanna.com/. Anna Sobaski is an Iowa City chef who has developed a line of excellent products that one can use to still have some familiar foods while maintaining a gluten-free diet. I'd still be cautious about how frequently to eat even gluten-free grains. More recipes for gluten-free living or vegan living, which is animal protein free, can be found at the following sites: http://www.vegan-food.net/; http://www.celiac.com; and http://www.glutenfreeda.com/index.asp.

© Gluten-free recipes from the Institute for Functional Medicine

The recipes marked by the © symbol are copyright and are used with permission granted by The Institute for Functional Medicine, 2009, www.functionalmedicine.org. No part of this content may be reproduced or transmitted in any form or by any means without the express written consent of The Institute for Functional Medicine, except as permitted by applicable law.

The Institute for Functional Medicine is an organization dedicated to training health care professionals about the core clinical imbalances that underlie various disease conditions. Those imbalances arise as environmental inputs, such as diet; nutrients (including air and water), exercise, and trauma are processed by one's body, mind, and spirit through a unique set of genetic predispositions, attitudes, and beliefs. The Institute for Functional Medicine has been very helpful in my journey to understanding my disease and developing my interventions.

Replacement guide

Milk
Rice, almond, coconut, or homemade nut milk (1/2 cup raw nuts or seeds with 1 cup water blended until smooth)

Cheese
Rice and almond brands; read labels and watch for casein-free brands

Eggs
Ener-G egg replacer or blend 1 tablespoon flaxseed with 1/4 cup water and allow to thicken

Peanut butter
Nut butters made from almonds, cashews, macadamia nuts, walnuts, pumpkin seeds, hazelnuts, or sesame (tahini)

Breading
Grind any allowable rice cracker and use as breading

Ice cream
Rice Dream (vanilla), Coconut Bliss™, berry sorbets

Soda
R.W. Knudsen seltzer and juice, water, diluted juice

Jams
Cascadian Farm®, Sorrel Ridge, Polaner (read label carefully)

Sugar
Agave syrup, fruit juice concentrate (Mystic Lake Dairy or Wax Orchard), brown rice syrup, stevia, honey, maple syrup, molasses

Pasta
Rice noodles (Tinkyada, Mrs. Leepers, Thai Life), 100% buckwheat udon noodles, cellophane noodles made from bean threads

Wheat bread
Rice cakes, rice crackers, rice almond and rice pecan breads, Ener-G brown rice or tapioca bread

Wheat cereals
Perky's Nutty Rice, crispy brown rice, puffed rice, puffed millet, cream of rice, quinoa flakes

Wheat flour
Rice, quinoa, amaranth, millet, teff, arrowroot, apioca bean; use nut and seed flours in combination with others to replace the full amount of wheat flour

* Foods rich in Omega-3 fatty acids
Omega-3 fatty acids are best absorbed by the body when eaten as food. Omega-3 fatty acids are present in:

Hemp and flax seed
Hemp and flax are both excellent sources of omega-3 fatty acids, although our bodies have to convert the omega-3 fatty acids into the form that is needed for cell membranes. We can convert approximately 40% of fish oil into the type of fatty acids our cell membranes need, but only about 10% of flax oil or hemp oil. They are also excellent sources of omega-9 fatty acids.

You can mix one part hemp nut butter or hemp seeds with three or four parts water in a high speed blender to make hemp milk. However, if you do the same with flax seeds you'll end with a gelatinous mess. You can grind flax seeds with a coffee grinder and add the flax meal to your casseroles, soups, or oatmeal.

However, do not use flax and hemp oils for frying, because the nutritious components will break down at high heat. Flax oil and hemp oil need to be kept in the refrigerator and in an opaque bottle, since light will also break down the oil.

You can use either flax oil or hemp oil in salad dressings. I have replaced olive oil with flax oil to create a variety of dressings that are very rich in omega-3 fatty acids. You can also use hemp oil as a substitute as well. Olive oil is high in omega-9 fatty acids, which are also good for you. But I generally use flax oil or hemp oil in my home-made dressings because, like many people, I could use more omega-3 fatty acids in my diet.

Very dark greens
Dark greens and algae are sources of omega-3 fatty acids.

Eggs
Eggs from chickens fed grass, crickets, or flax meal are good sources of omega-3 fatty acids. The egg carton will indicate if the nutrient is present.

Grass-fed animals
Grass-fed meat has a balanced ratio between omega-6 and omega-3 fatty acids. As such, it is much better for you to find a farmer who raises grass-

fed animals. Livestock that is "finished" with corn means the animal is NOT grass fed.

Fish

Fish, especially wild salmon, have high levels of omega-3s. The salmon must be wild-caught, not farmed, to be a good source. Canned wild salmon is less expensive than fresh or frozen wild salmon. Mackeral and herring are also rich sources of omega-3.

Mercury is a problem caused by the increasing amount of pollution in our waters. Many people avoid fish entirely for that reason. Alternatively, one can selectively eat types of fish with lower levels of mercury. An excellent resource for identifying the mercury levels in fish is located at the following Web site: http://www.nrdc.org/health/effects/mercury/guide.asp

Fish and seafood that typically have low levels of mercury:

Wild-caught: anchovy, catfish, clams, pacific cod, founder, haddock, herring, ocean perch, salmon, scallops, shrimps, and sole.

Farmed: oysters (except from the Gulf of Mexico), tilapia, and trout.

Fish and seafood that typically have high levels of mercury:

Atlantic: Pollack, cod, tuna, snapper, shark, orange roughy, swordfish. Gulf of Mexico: oysters, crab Southern Pacific: Chilean sea bass (Pantagonia toothfish).

† Foods rich in organic sulfur

Greens and cabbage
Kale, collards, and cabbage are all excellent sources of organic sulfur, which is necessary for the body to make GABA.

Mushrooms
Mushrooms are an excellent source of B vitamins and organic sulfur. As such, I like to have some mushrooms most every day. Shitake mushrooms are excellent and have a long history of medicinal use in China. But you

don't have to only eat the more exotic mushrooms for health benefits. The white button mushrooms common in American supermarkets are good for you, too.

If your family doesn't like mushrooms you can consider incorporating them into soups, gravies, and sauces after putting them through the blender. Otherwise, I'd simply add them to whatever else you are cooking that day. One of my favorite ways to enjoy mushrooms is to add them to bone broth and have mushroom soup. It's light and packed with tremendous nutrition.

‡ Antioxidant-rich foods

Foods that are brightly colored will be rich in antioxidants, including polyphenols, flavonoids, acanthocyanids (blue black), lutein (red), and caretnoids (yellow orange). Eating some of each color each day is preferable and would provide your mitochondria the much-needed variety of antioxidants for optimal health. These recipes give you just a small sample of ideas.

Aronia berries

I have become very fond of Aronia, which is a bush native to the Midwest. It is vigorous, tolerant of a wide range of soils, and is a heavy producer of black berries that ripen in September. They are approximately the size of cranberries. They are very tart and they have higher levels of antioxidants and resveratrol than blueberries. In fact, they have some of the highest antioxidant rating of any known berries, including the Acai berry.

One way to make eating so many fruit and vegetables easier and less costly is by having an edible landscape. Planting bushes that are decorative, produce fruit, and are easy to grow is one of the easiest ways to do this.

§ Bone and Joint Food

It is important that our bones and joints have a rich supply of calcium, magnesium, and other minerals to be healthy and strong. We need a lot of collagen, chondroitin, hyaline, and sulfur in the cartilage as well. Too many of us do not have adequate nutrition to maintain healthy joints. The consequence is early loss of cartilage in the knees and hips, leading to painful joints and, eventually, a joint replacement. Instead, try drinking a cup of bone broth prior to each meal to give your joints more of what they need.

Because many people with MS are often inactive, have sub-optimal magnesium intake, and poor vitamin-D levels, we are often at risk for fractures.

I encourage everyone to work on ensuring they get plenty of vitamin D3 (either through sunlight or supplements), plenty of calcium (through the cabbage family vegetables), and magnesium (through the bone broth).

Those who drink soda have a significant intake of acid. This acid leaches calcium from the teeth enamel and from the skeleton. The result is diffuse decay of the teeth, leading to rotten teeth, which eventually are either removed or capped. In addition, osteoporosis occurs at an early age, leading to fractures, which in the setting of multiple sclerosis leads to greater debility and disability. Elimination of soda is very important. In its place I suggest you drink iced tea. If it is too bitter for you, mix the tea with fruit juice of your choice. The tea/juice combination has numerous antioxidants and will be much healthier for your mitochondria and your bones.

Using bone broth as a soup base
Bone broth is full of glucosamine, collagen, and other micronutrients (e.g., minerals, vitamins, and amino acids) necessary for bone and joint health. It also provides a rich source of amino acids and minerals excellent for making neurotransmitters. You don't need to buy glucosamine. Drink bone broth instead of buying supplements. Have a cup of bone broth every day.

BEVERAGES

Americans purchase beverages with meals and throughout the day, which typically are filled with sugar and cream. Rarely do the beverages have any essential nutrients for our bodies. Water is usually a much healthier choice than the sugar or creamed beverages that we consume.

There are other, much healthier, options to consider. Instead of spending $3.00 or more on premium coffees and super-charged caffeine drinks, try making some of these beverages. If you need fast food you could make these smoothies for a quick, healthy breakfast. Or you could carry these with you for a quick healthy lunch.

Smoothies

Green tea, cocoa, ginger, cloves, cinnamon, and cardamom are all potent antioxidants. I combine these with hemp milk, which is made from hemp seeds and is an excellent source of omega-3 fatty acids and has all the essential amino acids. I do not need to use sugar, because the banana and spices reduce the bitterness considerably. These drinks are good cold or warm. I do not use cow's milk because some data suggests that diets high in dairy products produce a greater risk for MS. Instead, I use hemp milk and almond milk. This drink boosts antioxidant levels, omega-3 fatty-acid intake, and facilitates the brain's ability to make more GABA. All are good for brain health. I prefer to rotate my morning smoothies so that I do not have the same beverage each morning.

I enjoy cocoa and was initially without cocoa when I first gave up dairy. Then I discovered milk made with nuts. You can purchase ready-made hemp or almond milk in many large grocery stores and natural foods groceries. Alternatively, you can purchase hemp seeds and make your own hemp milk. Use one part hemp seeds and three parts water and run them through a high-speed blender. You can do the same with sesame seeds, almonds, filberts, or Brazil nuts. Or, you can take organic nut butter (smooth varieties) and mix with water in equal ratios. When blended with water, flax seeds make a more thickened, gelatinous drink, similar to adding psyllium seeds to water.

Cocoa Smoothie*‡

> 2 cups hemp milk (or soy or almond milk)
> 1 cup boiling water (or ice)
> 1 teaspoon unsweetened organic cocoa
> 1 – 2 teaspoons ground cinnamon
> 1 banana (fresh or frozen)
> ⅛ teaspoon algae (optional)
> ⅛ teaspoon dried kelp (optional)

Blend in a blender until frothy. If you are taking nutritional yeast or amino acid supplements, you can also add them to this smoothie. For a frozen drink use a frozen banana and ice cubes; for the hot drink use the fresh banana and hot water.

Power Sports Drink Smoothie‡

Ready-to-buy drinks with antioxidants, vitamins, and caffeine continue to grow in popularity – but why pay so much money for a product that is inferior to what you can so easily make at home? This "sports drink" supplies many antioxidants, vitamins, and minerals courtesy of the tea, ginger, and fruit juice. It also has some caffeine, which increases alertness, and theanine, which improves focus.

> 4 bags of green tea
> 3 cups of boiling water
> 1 to 2 slices of fresh ginger
> 3 cups of 100% fruit juice
> honey to taste (optional)

Brew 4 bags of green tea and the ginger using 3 cups of boiling water. Add fruit juice and honey, if desired. This drink may be served hot or cold.

Matcha (Green) Tea Smoothie‡

Matcha is a type of green tea where the dried, young tea leaves have been ground into a powder. It is the source of tea used for the Japanese tea ceremony. It is a terrific way to start your day. Finding a way to have your kids drink some green tea each day is an excellent way to help keep them focused and calmer. You can mix green tea into water, tofu, soymilk, juice, or coconut milk. I purchase green tea powder in bulk through the Internet and keep it in my freezer. To keep it affordable, instead of using a premium grade powdered tea, I use the less costly mixing grade for my smoothies. A couple of Web sites that sell green tea are: http://www.zenmatchatea.com/, http://www.matchasource.com/, and http://www.islandteashop.com/

>2 cups hemp milk (or soy or almond milk)
>1 cup boiling water (or ice)
>1 teaspoon Matcha green tea powder
>1–2 teaspoons ground cardamom or cinnamon
>1 banana (fresh or frozen)
>¼ teaspoon algae (optional)
>¼ teaspoon dried kelp (optional)

Blend in a blender until frothy. If you are taking nutritional yeast or amino acid supplements you can add them to the smoothie. Use a frozen banana and ice cubes to make a frozen version or hot water to make a hot version of this drink. Pineapple, pear, papaya, mango, or kiwi can be used for a more exotic flavor with the same health benefits.

Kale and Pear Smoothie†‡§

Dark leafy green kale is also packed with calcium in a form that the body finds easier to digest than milk—and that's a real bonus for your bones. Pair these nutritious but bitter leaves with pear, green grapes, an orange, and a banana, and you get a surprisingly sweet smoothie that is absolutely loaded with nutrition. These recipes are reproduced and reprinted with permission from Vitamix, Inc. The VitaMix Web site is an excellent source for recipes using vegetables and fruit.

> 1 cup green grapes
> 1 tablespoon lime or lemon juice
> ½ Bartlett pear
> 1 (120 g) banana, fresh or frozen
> 1 cup packed kale or collards
> ½ cup water
> 2 cups ice cubes

Place all ingredients into blender. Blend on high until smooth.

Leafy Green Smoothie†

This is an excellent way to get your kids to eat more greens. Gradually increase the amount of greens in the smoothie as they get familiar with the taste.

> 2 bananas
> 3 oranges, peeled, quartered
>   or 2 tablespoons lime or lemon juice
> 1 head romaine lettuce or spinach
> 4 cups cold water

Place all ingredients into blender. Blend on high until smooth.

Recipes

Parsley Greens Smoothie†

Parsley is packed with vitamins and minerals and is very inexpensive for the nutrition contained within them. If you are on a tight budget, parsley and green cabbage may be some of the best nutrition for your buck.

    1 cup of green grapes
    1 entire clump of parsley
    2 cups of water
    1 cup ice

Lime or lemon juice to taste to cut bitterness.
Mince parsley stems and leaves together. Combine with green grapes and place in blender with water and ice combination. Blend on high. Add the lime or lemon juice.

Aronia Smoothie‡

If you can't get Aronia berries in your area, you can substitute any kind of berries in this smoothie.

    ¼ cup Aronia berries
    3 cups soy, hemp, almond or other nut milk
    1 teaspoon cinnamon or cardamom

Place in a blender and blend on high until smooth. Serve immediately. Variation: Add one overripe banana.

Yerba Mate‡

Yerba Mate is a drink made from the leaves of a South American plant of the same name. It can be found in the herbal tea section of some grocery stores and natural foods stores. It is a great source of antioxidants. It contains approximately the same amount of caffeine as tea.

Brew it as you would coffee or tea and add honey to taste. Spices such as cinnamon, cardamom, cloves, and/or soy milk are good additions, too.

Ginger Tea‡

A couple slices of fresh ginger in hot water makes a refreshing tea. Ginger is a root traditionally used as a cooking and baking spice and as folk medicine for nausea. It is a great source of antioxidants and anti-inflammation nutrients.

Slicing ginger can be time-consuming, so an alternative is to chop ginger root with the blender, mixing it with lime or lemon juice. You can store the prepared ginger in a glass jar in the refrigerator. Mix a teaspoon or more with boiling water; add honey to taste.

Hibiscus Tea - Mukwa Juice‡

Hibiscus tea is a great source of the antioxidants acanthocyanids, polyphenols, and resveratrol.

    2 tablespoons Hibiscus Flowers
    4 cups water
    1 stick Cinnamon
    Honey to taste

Boil up to 2 hours. The used tea leaves (which are the flowers of the hibiscus) may be blended with a banana and milk for a smoothie later.

Turmeric Tea‡

Like ginger, turmeric is an excellent source of antioxidants and anti-inflammation nutrients. You have probably seen turmeric as a yellow-colored ground spice, alone or as a component in spice mixtures, such as mustard and curry. Fresh turmeric root may be difficult to find in a regular grocery store, but it can be found in many natural foods groceries and Asian grocery stores.

Turmeric tea can be prepared in the same manner as ginger tea. Chop or slice turmeric root and grind in the blender with lemon juice. Keep the resulting mixture in a glass jar in the refrigerator. You can mix with hot water according to how much spiciness you'd like in the tea.

Rooibus Tea ‡

Rooibus tea is not a true tea. It is an herb from South Africa where it has been noted to help sooth colicky babies, aid digestion, and help boost mood. Like green tea, rooibus is a great source of flavonols, polyphenols, quercetin, and minerals, including zinc, manganese. It is excellent hot or as an iced tea. Since it lacks caffeine it can be given to children. It can be used as a base for cooking as an alternative to water.

    1-2 tablespoons rooibus tea
    4 cups hot water
    1 stick Cinnamon
    Honey to taste

Let steep for 3 to 15 minutes. The more time spent steeping, the higher the level of antioxidants in the tea. This tea is also very nice mixed with fruit juice or with soy milk. As with the Hibiscus, the used tea leaves may be blended with a banana and milk for a smoothie later.

BREAKFAST AND BREAD

Baking Powder Biscuits©

    1¼ cups brown rice flour
    ½ cup tapioca flour
    ¼ cup ground flax seed
    4 teaspoons baking powder
    ¼ teaspoon salt
    3 tablespoons safflower or sesame oil
    1 cup applesauce, unsweetened

In a medium-large mixing bowl, stir together dry ingredients. Sprinkle oil on top and mix well with a pastry blender or fork, until consistency is crumbly. Mix in applesauce and stir until blended. Spoon heaping tablespoonfuls onto ungreased cookie sheet. With spoon, lightly shape into biscuit. Bake at 425 degrees for 15 to 18 minutes, until slightly browned. Serve warm for best flavor, but may be lightly reheated in a microwave. (Makes one dozen)

Pancakes or Flat Bread*

This is an excellent way to still let your family eat pancakes while you make the transition into gluten-free living. I routinely make extra pancakes, which I can then leave in the refrigerator to eat later in the week. The flax, chia, and hemp seeds are high-quality proteins and excellent sources of omega-3, omega-6, and omega-9 fatty acids. This is excellent nutrition and my kids love them, either as pancakes or made as flat bread to accompany a meal. Adding occasional meals that include gluten-free bread has made going gluten-free much easier for my kids. And I have found that I may have these twice a week without problem.

>   1 cup flax seed
>   1 cup gluten-free pancake mix
>   ½ cup chia seed (optional)
>   ¼ cup hemp seed
>   Coconut oil for the griddle
>   Non-dairy milk of choice

Grind the flax seed and chia seed in a coffee-grinder. If the hemp seed isn't already cracked, grind the hemp seeds. Mix the ground seeds with the gluten-free pancake mix. Stir in enough non-dairy milk to make a batter that pours easily.

Use coconut butter to grease the griddle. Turn the heat up to medium. When water sizzles when dropped onto the griddle, ladle the batter onto the griddle. Fry until the pancake is covered with tiny bubbles. Flip.

For the flatbread version, add less milk so the batter is stiff, like bread dough. Then roll out pieces of the dough to fry on a griddle as a gluten-free tortilla for a Mexican meal or as gluten-free Nan for an Indian meal.

Rice Pancakes©

1⅓ cups rice flour
½ cup oat flour
2 teaspoon baking powder
½ teaspoon baking soda
¼ teaspoon salt
2 tablespoon flax meal
    + 3 tablespoons boiling water
(egg replacement)
1 tablespoon coconut oil
1 tablespoon apple butter
1½ cups oat, almond, or rice milk, mixed with
    1½ tablespoon lemon juice (allow to sit 5 minutes until mixture curdles).

Mix dry ingredients and set aside. In large mixing bowl, beat apple butter, oil, egg-replacer, and milk. Add dry mixture and stir gently. Be careful not to over mix. Bake on preheated griddle. (Makes approximately 14 4-inch pancakes.)

French Toast©

1 cup soy milk
1-2 tablespoon ground flaxseed
2 tablespoons boiling water
½ teaspoon cinnamon
Stale rice bread

Mix the soymilk, flaxseed, water, and cinnamon. Dip stale rice bread into mixture and cook on preheated griddle greased with your choice of acceptable oil.

Whole-Grain Pancakes or Waffles©

2 cups any gluten-free flour combination
    (buckwheat, amaranth, rice, oat, etc.)
2 teaspoon baking powder
½ teaspoon baking soda
¼ teaspoon salt
2 tablespoon flax meal
    + 3 tablespoons boiling water
2 cups your choice: soy yogurt, fruit juice,
    milk (soy, almond, rice, or any milk soure
    with 2 teaspoon lemon juice until curdled)
1–2 tablespoons coconut oil
(3–4 tablespoon for waffles)

Mix dry ingredients and wet ingredients separately. Combine mixtures, stirring. Mixture will be a bit lumpy. Cook on preheated griddle or waffle iron. Serve with sautéed apples and cinnamon (recipe follows), unsweetened applesauce, or all-fruit syrup or pure maple syrup (in very small amounts). (Serves 4)

Granola©

4 cups rolled oats or
    other non-gluten-containing grain
½ –1 cup soy grits, optional (use only if
    soy is not a problem food)
1–2 cups sunflower seeds and chopped nuts
1 cup chopped dried fruit and chopped
    coconut (sugarless)
1 teaspoon cinnamon
½ cup honey or pure maple syrup
1 teaspoon vanilla
⅓ cup coconut oil

Combine dry and wet ingredients separately, and then stir both mixtures together. Bake at 325 degrees, stirring occasionally, until crunchy, about 2 1/2 hours.

Blueberry Banana Muffins©

⅔ cup mashed ripe banana
1 tablespoon flax meal
    + 2 tablespoons boiling water
½ cup oat, almond, or rice milk or apple juice
⅓ cup coconut oil (cold pressed preferred)
2 cups rice flour
1 teaspoon baking soda
1 teaspoon baking powder
1 cup fresh or frozen blueberries
¼ teaspoon salt

Beat together mashed banana and egg until creamy. Mix in milk and oil and beat well. Combine dry ingredients and add, stirring just until moistened. Gently mix in blueberries. Spoon batter into oiled and floured muffin pan, filling ⅔ full. Bake 15 minutes at 350 degrees or until lightly browned. (Makes 12 muffins)

Banana Breakfast Cake©

3 very ripe bananas, mashed
2 tablespoon lemon juice
¼ cup apple juice
⅓ cup coconut oil
1½ cup gluten-free flour mix
¼ teaspoon salt
½ teaspoon baking powder
½ teaspoon baking soda
½ cup oat bran
¾ cup raisins or currants

Mix mashed bananas and lemon juice until smooth. Stir in juice and oil. In a separate bowl, mix flour, salt, baking powder, and soda; mix in bran and add to bananas. Mix well and stir in raisins. Batter will be stiff. Spoon into oiled 8-by-8-inch square pan. Bake at 350 degrees for 35 to 40 minutes. Cool on rack. Cut into squares. Freezes well in individual baggies for lunch-box treats. (Makes 9 squares)

Gluten-Free Muesli©

3 cups puffed rice
2 cups crispy brown rice cereal
2 cups puffed millet
1 cup sliced almonds
1 cup sunflower seeds
1½ cups of any combination of the following dried fruit bits:
     currants, dates, cherries, apples, peaches, or apricots

Combine all ingredients and store in airtight container. Can be used as a breakfast cereal or portable snack. Also used in Muesli Cookies recipe, below. (Makes 10 cups)

Muesli Cookies©

2 cups muesli
⅓ cup brown rice syrup or honey
2 tablespoon coconut oil (cold pressed)
½ cup ripe banana, mashed

Mix ingredients well and drop by rounded tablespoons on a greased cookie sheet 1 inch apart. Bake at 350 degrees for 30 to 35 minutes.

Rice Cereal Crispies©

> 1 teaspoon coconut oil
> ½ cup brown rice syrup
> 2 tablespoon sesame tahini
> (or other nut butter)
> 1 tablespoon vanilla extract
> 2 cups crispy brown rice cereal, 1 cup each puffed rice and puffed millet, and 2 cups Perky's Nutty Rice (or use only 6 cups of crispy brown rice or any combination of gluten-free cereals)
> ½ cup sunflower seeds
> ½ cup currants, chopped dried apple, or dates

In large pot, over low heat, stir oil, rice syrup, and tahini until bubbly; remove from heat and stir in vanilla. Add remaining ingredients and mix until "well acquainted" with a wooden spoon. Press into ungreased 13-by-9-inch pan. It will set in 30 minutes at room temperature. Cut into squares and store in an airtight container, not refrigerated. (Makes 2 dozen squares)

APPETIZERS

Salmon Dip for Vegetables*

Wild salmon is rich in omega-3 fatty acids, but farmed salmon is not. Use canned wild salmon to make a pleasant dip or sandwich spread.

  1 can wild salmon
  ½ stalk celery, chopped
  1 green onion, sliced
  ¼ pound silken or soft tofu, mashed
  1 tablespoon nut butter
      (such as almond, hemp, or cashew)

Mix and season to taste.

Greens as a Wrap†§

You can use steamed collards or kale as a wrap. Place a spoon of cooked beans or a mixture of rice and meat. Then cover with a red sauce (or salsa or coconut milk) and bake at 350 degrees for 30 minutes. We have used canned wild salmon which was mixed with chopped onions, celery, flax oil and brewer's yeast as the filling with lightly steamed collard greens wrap was another big hit at our house.

Kale Chips†‡§

Kale recipes aren't normally on the top of most parents lists when they're looking for vegetables the kids will like. But I urge you to try this crispy kale. It is really extraordinary. Although the kale is roasted, not fried, it becomes crispy and salty, almost like French fries. Cooking with olive oil and shallot softens kale's native bitterness.

> 6-8 cups chopped fresh kale,
>   hard stems removed
> 2 tablespoon olive oil
> 1 teaspoon apple cider vinegar
> ½ teaspoon kosher salt or sea salt

Place a rack on the lowest shelf of your oven. Preheat oven to 350 degrees F. Spread kale out on a sturdy baking sheet. Drizzle with olive oil and apple cider vinegar. Toss to coat completely. Place on the lowest rack of the oven and bake for 10 minutes.

   Remove from oven and stir so that kale can get crispy all over. Bake another 8 to 12 minutes, or until kale is crispy. It should be just lightly browned and crispy to the touch. If kale still bends, rather than crackles, when you touch it, it isn't done yet. Return it to the oven. Turn down the heat if it is getting too brown. Continue cooking until crispy. Remove from oven and sprinkle with sea salt.

Oven-Baked Fries©

Spray a large cookie sheet with olive oil. Slice a combination of white and sweet potatoes into French fry slices and put on cookie sheet in a single layer. Spray with more olive oil. Bake at 400 degrees for about 30 to 45 minutes (time depends on the size of your slices). For a crispy taste, turn oven to broil broil potatoes for about 3 to 5 minutes.

Walnut Spread©

    15-oz. can garbanzo beans
    1 cup chopped walnuts
    1 cup lightly packed fresh basil leaves
    ¼ cup olive oil
    2 tablespoons lemon juice
    ¼ teaspoon each salt and pepper

Drain beans, reserving liquid. In food processor, combine ¼ cup reserved liquid with remaining ingredients. Cover and process, scraping down sides and adding liquid as needed to make a smooth mixture. Store in refrigerator for 4 to 5 days. Serve with rice crackers and/or raw baby carrots, cucumber sticks, and fresh string beans (or any raw veggie you like). (Yields 2.5 cups)

Marinated Veggies©‡†

    ½ cup olive oil
    ¼ cup balsamic vinegar (any vinegar is fine,
        balsamic is very full-flavored)
    1 teaspoon each dried oregano and basil
        or 2 tablespoons chopped fresh
    2 cloves garlic, slivered
    ½ teaspoon salt
    1 can artichoke hearts in water,
        cut in halves or quarters
    1 can hearts of palm, cut into ¼-inch slices
    1 can pitted black olives
    ½ pound of mushrooms,
        cleaned and quartered

Mix marinade ingredients in a jar. Mix veggies in a bowl and pour marinade over. Marinate 8 to 24 hours, tossing frequently. Serve with toothpicks. Leftover marinade can be used as salad dressing.

DRESSINGS AND SAUCES

Basic Flax / Hemp Oil Dressing — Version 1*

Equal parts of:

> Flax or hemp oil
> Soy sauce
> Rice vinegar

Basic Flax / Hemp Oil Dressing — Version 2*

Equal parts of:

> Flax / hemp oil
> Rice vinegar
>
> ½ as much concentrated cherry
> or blueberry juice

Basic Flax / Hemp Oil Dressing — Version 3*

Equal parts of:

> Flax / hemp oil
> Fresh basil
> Pine nuts
> Rice vinegar
>
> Garlic to taste
> Finely minced ginger root to taste

Mix the ingredients together in a blender or a jar with a lid and shake vigorously. Remember that the oil is fragile. You'll need an opaque jar and to refrigerate the dressings.

Absolutely Fabulous Greek/House Dressing*

¼ cup plus 2 teaspoons flax or hemp oil
¾ teaspoon garlic powder
¾ teaspoon dried oregano
¾ teaspoon dried basil
½ teaspoon pepper
½ teaspoon salt
½ teaspoon onion powder
½ teaspoon Dijon-style mustard
⅓ cup plus 1 tablespoon red wine vinegar

In a very large container, mix together the oil, garlic powder, oregano, basil, pepper, salt, onion powder, and Dijon-style mustard. Pour in the vinegar, and mix vigorously until well blended. Store tightly covered at room temperature.

Cranberry Vinaigrette*‡

You can use any fruit juice concentrate of your choice to make other vinaigrettes, such as raspberry or blueberry.

1½ tablespoons flax or hemp oil
1 tablespoon frozen cranberry-juice
        concentrate, thawed
1 tablespoon rice-wine vinegar
1 teaspoon Dijon mustard
Salt and freshly ground pepper, to taste

Combine all ingredients in a glass jar with a tight-fitting lid and shake until well blended.

Cilantro-Lime Salad Dressing*

    1 cup flax or hemp oil
    1 bunch cilantro
    1 clove garlic
    2 green onions
    Salt and freshly ground pepper, to taste

Combine all ingredients in a glass jar with a tight-fitting lid and shake until well blended.

Tahini Dressing©

    ½ cup flax oil, hemp oil or extra-virgin
        or light olive oil
    ¼ cup sesame tahini
    2 to 3 tablespoons apple cider vinegar
    1 lemon (juiced)
    2 tablespoons reduced sodium
        natural soy sauce
    2 tablespoons water
    1 teaspoons dried dill
    1 teaspoons dried chives, optional
    Mixed greens

Combine all ingredients in a bottle with a tight lid and shake well. Pour over salad greens and veggies; toss well. Will keep for up to 2 weeks, refrigerated. Shake before each use. (Serves 12)

Vinaigrette Dressing©

Note: Ingredient amounts in this recipe are approximate—use more or less of certain ingredients to adapt recipe to your personal taste.

> ¼ cup each flax and extra-virgin olive oils
> 3 tablespoons balsamic vinegar
> > (preferred because it has the
> > richest flavor)
> 2–3 tablespoons water
> 1 teaspoon dry mustard
> 1–3 cloves garlic (whole pieces
> > for flavor or crushed for stronger taste)
> Salt and pepper to taste
> Oregano, basil, parsley, tarragon,
> > or any herbs of your choice, fresh or dried

Place vinegar, water, and mustard in a tightly capped jar and shake well to thoroughly dissolve mustard. Add oil and remaining ingredients and shake well again. Store refrigerated and shake well before using. Dressing will harden when cold; allow 5 to10 minutes to reliquify. (Serves 6)

Cranberry Mole‡

Making mole (a traditional Mexican sauce) doesn't have to be an all-day process, and eating it doesn't have to be a dietary nightmare, especially if you use sweet cranberries for flavor, cut down on the oil, and reduce the huge quantity of nuts and seeds often used. This recipe makes more than you may need for Thanksgiving dinner, but the leftovers are delicious on Southwestern-style turkey sandwiches or quesadillas (being careful to use gluten-free bread or tortillas).

     5 cups water
     10 dried chilies, any combination of
             New Mexico, pasilla and/or ancho
             (see Ingredient notes)
     ½ cup dried cranberries
     4 tomatillos, papery husks removed,
             rinsed and halved (see Ingredient notes)
     2 plum tomatoes, halved
     ¼ cup sliced almonds
     1 teaspoon olive oil
     1 small, very ripe, almost black plantain,
             (about 10 ounces), peeled and thinly sliced
             (see Ingredient notes)
     3 cloves garlic, peeled and halved
     2 teaspoons ground cinnamon
     ¼ teaspoon ground allspice
     ¼ teaspoon ground cloves
     2 cups bone chicken broth
     1 ounce bittersweet chocolate, grated
     ½ teaspoon salt
     ¼ teaspoon freshly ground pepper

Bring water to a boil in a medium saucepan. Stem and seed chilies, then tear the skins into large chunks. Place the chilies and dried cranberries in a large bowl; cover with boiling water. Set aside to soften.

Position rack at top level of oven; preheat broiler. Lightly oil a large baking sheet with a rim. Place tomatillos and tomatoes cut-side down on the baking sheet. Broil until the skins char, about 6 minutes. Transfer the

92

tomatillos, tomatoes, and any juices to a food processor or blender.

Meanwhile, toast almonds in a dry medium skillet over medium heat, stirring, until lightly browned, about 4 minutes. Transfer to the food processor or blender. Heat oil in the same pan over medium heat. Add plantain and cook until lightly browned, 4 to 5 minutes, turning the slices once. Transfer to the food processor or blender.

Place garlic in the same pan over medium-low heat; cook, stirring occasionally, just until golden, about 3 minutes. Add to the food processor or blender. Drain the chilies and cranberries; transfer to the food processor or blender. Add cinnamon, allspice, and cloves. Process until smooth, scraping down the sides as necessary, about 3 minutes.

Pour the puree into a large saucepan. Stir in broth, chocolate, salt, and pepper. Cook over medium-high heat, stirring constantly, until the mole begins to bubble, 3 to 4 minutes. Reduce heat and gently simmer, stirring constantly, until the mole is steaming and slightly thickened, about 10 minutes.

Cranberry-Grape Relish‡

This is an excellent sweet-tart accompaniment for turkey or other poultry or meat dishes. One could replace the cranberries with Aronia berries as an alternative to the cranberries. If you use grapes with seeds and put them through a high-speed blender, then you retain the potent antioxidants that are found in the grape seeds. Notably, grape seed extract is sold as a supplement because it is beneficial for lowering cholesterol, raising the food cholesterol (HDL), and lowering inflammation in the body.

> ½ pound seedless green grapes, stemmed
>   (2 cups)
> ¼ cup dried cranberries
> ¼ cup dry white wine
> ¼ cup orange juice
> 1½ tablespoons honey
> 1 tablespoon lime juice

Combine all ingredients in a saucepan. Bring to a boil over medium heat. Cook, stirring frequently, until thickened, 30 to 35 minutes. Serve warm or cold.

Cranberry Sauce with Cherries, Marsala, and Rosemary‡

This is wonderful with pork or turkey. It can be prepared a week ahead. Cover and keep refrigerated. I usually make at least a double recipe of this and freeze it so we can enjoy it most of the year. The fresh rosemary, chopped very fine, is important, so don't leave that out. Enjoy!

½ cup dried tart cherries
12-oz bag fresh cranberries
12-oz bag frozen dark sweet cherries
(about 2⅔ cups)
1 cup (packed) golden brown sugar
1 teaspoon minced fresh rosemary
½ teaspoon ground allspice
½ cup of Marsala wine

Combine Marsala and dried cherries in a deep saucepan. Boil until mixture is reduced to ⅔ cup, about 8 minutes. Mix in remaining ingredients. Bring to boil, stirring occasionally. Reduce heat to medium, cover pan, and simmer, stirring occasionally, until cranberries burst and mixture thickens, about 8 minutes. Transfer to bowl. Refrigerate until cold, about 3 hours.

Spicy Cranberry Chutney‡

What could be better with a simple roast or grilled vegetables than a spicy fruit chutney? Nothing, except knowing it was a gift from someone you cherish. Consider giving with a decorative serving spoon tied to the side of the jar with raffia.

> 8 cups fresh or frozen cranberries, (2 pounds)
> 2 shallots, minced
> 2 jalapeno peppers, seeded and minced
> 2 cloves garlic, minced
> 1½ cups packed light brown sugar
> 1½ cups granulated sugar
> ½ cups red-wine vinegar
> 2 tablespoons minced fresh ginger
> 2 tablespoons whole mustard seeds
> 1 tablespoon freshly grated orange zest
> 1 tablespoon freshly grated lemon zest
> 2 teaspoons salt

Combine all ingredients in a large saucepan; bring to a boil over high heat. Simmer, uncovered, stirring often, until the cranberries have broken down and the mixture has thickened somewhat, 10 to 15 minutes. Let cool completely. Ladle the chutney into clean jars and refrigerate.

SALADS

Edamame, Asparagus, and Arugula Salad©†

½ lb. medium asparagus, ends trimmed
2 cups shelled frozen edamame, defrosted
2 tablespoons extra-virgin olive oil, divided
½ lb. arugula, coarse stems discarded
¼ cup Brewer's yeast
2 teaspoons balsamic vinegar

Cut trimmed asparagus stalks into ¼-inch slices on a diagonal, leaving 1 inch tips to reserve as garnish. Blanche tips in a 3-quart pot of water for 1 minute only. Remove from water. Toss edamame with blanched asparagus tips and raw sliced stalks with 1 tbs. olive oil and salt and pepper to taste. Pile arugula in a salad bowl and toss with remaining 1 tbs. olive oil and salt and pepper to taste. Top arugula with veggies and sprinkle Brewer's yeast. Drizzle with vinegar. (Serves 4)

Greek Mushroom Salad©†

1 tablespoon hemp or flax oil
½ lb. mushrooms
3 cloves garlic, chopped fine
1 teaspoon both basil and marjoram
1 medium tomato, diced
3 tablespoons lemon juice
½ cup water
1 pinch salt
1 pinch fresh ground pepper
1 tablespoon fresh chopped parsley or fresh cilantro

Heat the oil on low in a frying pan, then gently sauté the mushrooms for 2 to 3 minutes. Do not overcook. Sprinkle in garlic and basil, then stir-fry for a minute or two until mushrooms are well coated. Add the tomato, lemon juice, water, salt, and pepper. Stir together and cook until the tomato softens. Remove from heat and let cool. Garnish with chopped herbs. (Serves 6)

Quinoa Salad©‡

> 3 cups water or chicken or vegetable broth
> 1½ cups quinoa, well rinsed
>   (will taste bitter if not well rinsed)
> 1 cup fresh or frozen peas (baby peas
>   are best, just defrosted)
> Any leftover veggie you like—be creative (broccoli, asparagus, green
>   beans, etc.)
> 1 chopped red onion
> 1 red pepper, chopped
> 1 cup cherry tomatoes
> ½ cup chopped black olives, optional
> ½ cup hemp or flax oil
> 2–3 tablespoons balsamic vinegar
>   or lemon juice
> 1–2 cloves garlic, crushed
> 2–4 tablespoons fresh dill, chopped or
>   1 tablespoon dried
> 2 tablespoons chopped fresh parsley

Bring 3 cups water or broth to a boil. Add rinsed quinoa and bring back to boil. Simmer uncovered for about 15 minutes until liquid is well absorbed. Transfer to large bowl and allow to cool with a small amount of olive oil stirred in to prevent sticking. While cooling, mix together remaining oil, vinegar or lemon juice, dill, and garlic in a small bowl. Add to quinoa with remaining ingredients when cool and toss well. Chill before serving. (Serves 8 to 10)

Cabbage Salad©‡†

1 small to medium head red cabbage, thinly sliced (or use half red and half green cabbage)
8 sliced radishes or 1 grated carrot
3 green apples, diced
1 stalk celery, chopped
½ cup chopped walnuts or pecans
Dash garlic powder
2 tablespoons hemp oil
2 teaspoons vinegar
1 teaspoon lemon juice

Mix all ingredients in a bowl and allow to sit for an hour, stirring once or twice. Serve cold or at room temperature. (Serves 4 to 6)

Fruity Spinach Salad©‡†

1 lb. fresh spinach, washed, dried, torn into pieces
1 pint fresh organic strawberries or raspberries, washed
½ cup chopped walnuts or sliced almonds

Dressing:

2 tablespoons sesame seeds
1 tablespoon poppy seeds
2 scallions, chopped
¼ cup flaxseed oil
¼ cup safflower oil
¼ cup balsamic vinegar

Cut berries in half and arrange over spinach in serving bowl. Combine dressing ingredients in blender or food processor and process until smooth. Just before serving, pour over salad and toss. Garnish with nuts. (Serves 6 to 8)

Red Root Salad‡

This has been a big hit at our house and is a rich source of antioxidants and other phytonutrients good for your mitochondria.

Red beets
Yellow beets
Parsnips
Carrots
Rutabaga
Turnips
2 stalks celery
½ to 1 inch grated ginger

Dressing

1 tablespoon each of flax oil,
rice vinegar, soy sauce.

Grate any combination of the above roots in approximately equal proportions Add minced celery in equal proportion to the red beets. Add orange zest (grated from the skin of an orange). Finely chop the orange or simply squeeze for the juice. Add fresh ginger finely minced or grated. If the salad seems bitter you can add more soy sauce.

Kale or Collard Greens Ginger Salad†‡§

Many people are put off by the bitter taste of plain kale. This can be entirely resolved by complementing the flavor with the addition of fruit. Since kale and collard greens are such an excellent source of many potent intracellular antioxidants and amino acids, it is well worth the effort to find recipes you and your family will enjoy.

> 1 head of kale or collard greens
> 4 cloves of garlic minced or 1 small onion chopped
> ½ to 1 inch of grated ginger root
> 3 to 6 oranges
> ¼ to ½ cups of dried cranberries
> ¼ cup sesame seeds
> Dressing (choice of dressing from above recipes)

Mince garlic or onions; sit for 15 minutes to allow the nutrients to stabilize prior to use. When the garlic/onions are cut across, a reaction occurs that stabilizes the micronutrients, which allows them to not be lost in cooking or in the marinade.

To cut the greens, use the chiffonade technique to cut the leaves into long thin strips. Roll up a couple leaves of kale or collard greens into a cylinder shape and slice across the 'barrel' to get thin 1/4 to 1/2 inch wide strips.

Cut up citrus (any combination of pink grapefruit, orange, lemon, or lime is excellent) into small bite-size pieces. Add dried cranberries and sesame seeds.

Marinade the greens with your choice of dressing for at least one hour prior to serving.

Carrot Salad©‡

     2 cups shredded carrot
     ½ cup diced celery
     ¼ cup sunflower seeds
     3–4 tablespoon hemp or flax oil
     2 tablespoon pineapple juice

Mix all ingredients and chill for several hours before serving. (Serves 4)

SOUPS AND STEWS

Homemade Bone Broth§

Save chicken bones from your meals and use them to make chicken broth. Save bones from your pork chops, ribs, or any soup bones. You can also use mussel or clam shells to make broth.

The vinegar helps draw the minerals out of the bone (magnesium, calcium, zinc, boron, and others). The seaweed provides an excellent of source of iodine and other trace minerals to your broth and will not add a noticeable seaweed flavor. (In fact, when I began adding the dried seaweed my family told me the broth was especially good. I took that as a sign their bodies appreciated the additional trace minerals that came with the seaweed. I've been adding it ever since.)

> Bones, saved from previous cooking
> Scraps of vegetables, such as celery, parsley, and any vegetable
>   that looks "past its prime"
> Large stock pot or soup pot half full of water
> 2 to 4 tablespoons of vinegar
> 1 tablespoon dried powdered kelp or dulse, or part of a whole leaf
> 1 packet gelatin

Put all ingredients except seaweed and gelatin into the pot and simmer for 2 or more hours (ideally 24 hours). Add water if needed. Strain out the vegetables and bones and discard them. Dissolve a packet of plain gelatin in the broth. Freeze it in pint or quart batches for future use.

I leave one or two cups in the refrigerator to gently sauté vegetables in homemade broth. Because the broth has just a small amount of fat, sautéing with broth provides the benefits of sauté without the calories of using frying oil. Put three tablespoons in a pan whenever you wish to sauté or stir-fry fresh vegetables. That'll give you that stir-fry taste without losing the antioxidant capabilities in the food you're cooking!

Onion Mushroom Soup§†

    1 onion
    2 to 3 garlic
    1 cup mushrooms
    1 to 3 teaspoons dried kelp or dulse
    3 cups bone broth or more

Mince the garlic and chop the onions. Let broth sit for fifteen minutes prior to cooking. That is because the important sulfur compounds will stabilize once the garlic or onion have been cut up. This allows more nutrients to be retained after cooking.

Wipe off the mushrooms and cut up into bite-size pieces. Add the mushrooms and onions to the chicken broth. Cook gently until the onions are translucent. Add the tamari sauce and increase to taste (as opposed to adding salt).

It adds a tremendous number of important bone and cartilage nutrients to your diet!

An excellent variation is to add 1 to 3 cups of parsley or cilantro juice just prior to serving. Blend a whole bunch of greens with 3 cups of water on high until smooth. Add to soups just prior to serving to taste.

Wild Rice Cranberry Soup§‡

The tart berries offer a wonderful contrast to the broth. Feel free to add any leftover vegetables you have on hand. Save the bones from your holiday turkey for bone broth and chop the leftover meat to add to soups. Add a salad of green leaves and you have a meal that is rich in sulfur and anti-oxidants and, if you had seaweed in the bone broth, it is loaded with iodine and trace minerals.

⅓ cup wild rice
2 to 4 cups bone broth
1 chopped onion
2 minced garlic cloves
1 sliced onion
1 sliced carrots
1 cup mixture of aronia and/or cranberries
2 cups soy milk or other nut milk or coconut milk
1 cup chopped turkey or chicken

Simmer the wild rice, garlic, onions, and mushrooms in the bone broth for twenty minutes. Then add the sliced carrots and simmer another 15 minutes. Just prior to serving stir in the soy milk and turkey. Serve immediately.

Fish Chowder*‡†

My daughter made this wonderful chowder at a friend's house. The original recipe called for cream and white potatoes. I replaced the cream with coconut milk and added yam. With all of the fish, mushrooms, onions, and garlic, it is filled with organic sulfur. Yams are a rich source of antioxidants.

  2 onions, minced
  4 cloves garlic, minced
  4 cans clam juice
  1 sweet potato or yam, diced
  2-3 small red potatoes
  ½ cup minced parsley leaves
  1 cup chopped mushrooms
  1 can of coconut milk
  2 pounds cod or other fish, cut into mouth-sized pieces

Sauté onions and mushrooms in 1 to 2 tablespoons of water or broth until onions are translucent. Then add clam juice and coconut milk. Bring to a simmer and add diced yam and potatoes. Simmer approximately 15 minutes until almost done. Add fish and simmer another 5 minutes. Do not overcook the fish. Stir in fresh parsley just before serving.

Bouillabaisse*§

My kids love bouillabaisse. According to tradition, there should be at least five different kinds of fish in a proper bouillabaisse. Use as many different types of fish as you can, such as flounder, haddock, cod, perch, white fish, whiting, porgies, bluefish, or bass — almost any combination works. Count on at least three kinds of fish if you want enough for six servings. I make it up to the point where I'd be ready to add the fish or shellfish. I then split my batch. Half I freeze in one-quart containers. The other half I continue and add the fish and shellfish. I do this because reheating the fish gives it a rubbery consistency.

> 1-2 pounds of oysters, clams, or mussels
> 1 cup cooked shrimp, crab, or lobster meat, or rock lobster tails
> 1-2 pounds of scallops, cod, salmon, or other fish
> 2 thinly sliced onions
> 2 or 3 leeks, thinly sliced
> 2 cloves garlic, crushed
> 1 large tomato, chopped, or 1 can chopped tomatoes
> 1 sweet red pepper, chopped
> 3 sprigs fresh thyme or 3/4 teaspoon dried thyme
> 1 bay leaf
> 2-3 whole cloves
> Zest of an orange, with the orange chopped
> ¼ teaspoon powdered saffron
> 2 teaspoons salt
> ¼ teaspoon freshly ground black pepper
> 2 cans of clam juice or fish broth
> 2 tablespoons lemon juice
> ⅔ cup white wine

Heat ¼ cup of the olive oil in a large (6-qt) saucepan. When it is hot, add onions and shallots (or leeks). Sauté for a minute, then add crushed garlic (more or less to taste) and sweet red pepper. Add tomato, celery, and fennel. Stir the vegetables into the oil with a wooden spoon until well coated. Then add another ¼ cup of olive oil, thyme, bay leaf, cloves, and the orange zest. Cook until the onion is soft and golden but not brown. Add saffron, salt, pepper. Add clam juice, chopped orange, and lemon juice and simmer for 15 minutes. This where I decide to split my batch and freeze some broth or consider whether we can eat the whole batch.

Cut fish fillets into 2-inch pieces. Add the pieces of fish and 2 cups of water to the vegetable mixture. Simmer, uncovered, for about 5 minutes so you do not overcook the fish. Add oysters, clams, or mussels (though these may be omitted if desired) and shrimp, crabmeat, or lobster tails, cut into pieces or left whole, and white wine. If the shellfish has already been cooked, all you need to do is bring the bouillabaisse back to a simmer. Do not overcook or the fish will become rubbery. Serve as soon as it begins to simmer.

Black Collards or Kale Soup †§

This is an extremely simple winter soup that will bring warmth and over-tones of happiness to the kitchen. My friend Sharon provided the recipe, simply listing ingredients; I have given amounts but feel free to adjust them to suit your taste.

    1-2 pounds of finely sliced collards or kale
    A medium sized onion, minced
    2 cloves garlic, crushed
    A medium carrot, minced
    A stalk of celery, minced
    A sprig of fresh thyme
    1 inch of grated ginger
    1 can crushed tomatoes
    2 small red potatoes diced
    Salt and pepper to taste
    2 quarts simmering bone broth

Mince the garlic, chop the onion, and slice greens into 1/4 inch strips; let sit for 15 minutes. Mince carrot and celery and dice potatoes. Cook onion, carrot, celery, and garlic in 1/2 cup of bone broth until the onion is translucent. Add the remainder of the broth, thyme, ginger, potatoes, greens, and tomatoes. Simmer the soup for an hour.

Creamy Greens Soup†§

Turmeric goes beautifully with greens. You can add a bit of red pepper flake to make this as spicy as you like. If you have gluten-free bread, this makes a wonderful meal.

> ½ cup lentils
> ½ cup brown rice, wild rice or quinoa
> ½ medium onion, finely chopped
> 2 garlic cloves
> 4 tablespoon bone broth to sauté onion
> 2 pounds greens (collards, kale or other dark greens)
> 5 cups bone broth

> Spices

> 1 teaspoon of cumin powder
> ½ to 1 teaspoon of curry powder
> 1 teaspoon of sea salt, to taste

Tahini Dressing

> 1 tablespoon tahini or other nut butter of choice
> 2 tablespoons flax oil
> Bragg's Liquid Aminos (lower in sodium and also gluten free)
>   or soy sauce to taste

Prior to cooking, add all spices together in a small bowl and mix well (this prevents clumping when added to the cooking pot later). Wash greens and chop finely; let sit 10 minutes. Mince garlic, chop onions, and let sit 10 minutes. Using 1/2 cup bone both, sauté the onion and garlic. When onions are translucent, stir in the spices. Then stir in the lentils and rice/quinoa right away. Puree in a blender. Mix the soup with the tahini dressing really well. Serves 2 hungry adults.

Split Pea Soup©

> 3 cups dry split peas, well rinsed
> 2 quarts water
> 1 bay leaf
> 1 large onion, finely chopped
> 2 cloves garlic, minced
> 3 stalks celery, chopped
> 3 medium carrots, sliced
> Salt and black pepper to taste
> 2 tablespoon apple cider vinegar or rice vinegar
> Ham, or other meat according to preferences

Place split peas, water, and bay leaf in Dutch oven. Bring to boil and lower heat to simmer, partially covered, for about 20 minutes. Add vegetables and simmer, partly covered, for about 40 minutes, stirring occasionally. Add more water as needed. Add pepper, salt, and vinegar to taste. (Serves 6)

Autumn Bean Soup©‡

    2 cups white kidney beans (cannellini); include any liquid
           from canned beans
    1–2 cups kidney or red beans (canned or cooked from dry)
    1½–2 cups chickpeas (garbanzos, canned or cooked from dry)
    2–3 cups fresh spinach or escarole, washed, drained,
           and chopped or 10 oz. frozen chopped spinach
    4 cups chicken broth (read ingredients to be sure it is gluten free)
    2 onions, chopped
    1 large clove garlic, minced
    1 teaspoon dried basil
    1 tablespoon dried parsley
    1 teaspoon dried oregano
    Pepper to taste
    Brewer's yeast for garnish, optional

Combine all ingredients and simmer until onions are soft, about 45 minutes. Serve immediately, garnished with Brewer's yeast, if desired. Substitute bone broth for the chicken broth for a boost for your bones. (Serves 6)

Asian Gazpacho©‡

6 tomatoes, seeded and finely chopped or 1 28-oz. can
      chopped tomatoes
2 cups vegetable broth
1 teaspoon dry sherry
2 tablespoons chopped fresh cilantro
1 tablespoon light soy sauce
4 scallions, white part only
4 thin slivers of fresh ginger
½ teaspoon Chinese chili sauce, to taste
2 limes

Place the tomatoes, over low heat, in a 2- or 3-quart saucepan. Add vegetable broth, sherry, cilantro, soy sauce, scallions, and ginger. Bring to a simmer and cook for 20 minutes. Remove from heat and allow to cool for a few minutes. Puree in a food processor or blender. Chill. Just before serving, stir in chili sauce. Grate the peel of one lime and add to the soup. Squeeze the juice from both limes into the soup. (Serves 6)

Creamy Cold Tomato Soup©‡

1 cucumber, chopped
1 scallion, chopped
1 clove garlic
4 cups tomato juice
1 cup soft tofu
1 green pepper, chopped
½ teaspoon dill weed
Sliced mushrooms or tomato chunks for garnish

Combine all ingredients (except tofu) in small amounts in blender and blend until smooth. Use salt sparingly, if needed, and pepper. Whisk in tofu. Chill several hours before serving and garnish as desired with mushrooms or tomato. (Serves 5)

Lentil Soup©‡

    2 cloves garlic, minced
    1 medium onion, chopped
    2 large carrots, sliced or chopped
    2 stalks celery, chopped
    1 ½ cups red and/or green lentils, well rinsed
    2 quarts water or broth
    Pinch thyme or any herbs of your choice
    Salt to taste

Combine first 6 ingredients and bring to boil. Add seasonings. Reduce heat to medium-low and simmer, partially covered, until lentils are soft. Green lentils need about 45 minutes to 1 hour, while red lentils only need 20 to 30 minutes. Puree half of the soup in the blender if you prefer a creamy soup. (Serves 4) (Use bone broth for a boost for your bones.)

Quinoa Vegetable Soup©‡

    4 cups water or bone broth
    ¼ cup quinoa, well rinsed
    ½ cup carrots, diced
    ¼ cup celery, diced
    2 tablespoons onion, chopped
    ¼ cup green pepper, diced
    2 cloves garlic, chopped
    1 teaspoons olive oil
    ½ cup tomatoes, chopped
    ½ cup cabbage, chopped
    1 teaspoon salt
    Parsley, chopped

Sauté quinoa, carrots, celery, onions, green pepper, and garlic in oil until golden brown. Add water, tomatoes, and cabbage and bring to a boil. Simmer 20 to 30 minutes, or until tender. Season to taste and garnish with parsley. For variations, try adding some of your other favorite vegetables, chopped and sautéed. (Serves 4 to 6)

Curried Cream of Broccoli Soup©‡

    1 tablespoon olive oil
    1 small onion, finely chopped
    2 teaspoons curry powder
    ¼ teaspoon powdered cumin
    1 bunch broccoli, trimmed and chopped (may substitute
        2 packages frozen chopped
    2 cups chicken broth or bone broth
    2 cups water
    1 can coconut milk
    Salt and pepper to taste

Heat oil in soup pot and sauté onion in it with curry and cumin until limp. Add broccoli, stock, and water. Simmer, covered, until tender (about 15 minutes). Add coconut milk to soup. If you prefer, you may blend the whole soup, leaving a few whole pieces of broccoli for garnish. Reheat, but do not boil. Cauliflower may be combined with broccoli for a different flavor. (Serves 4 to 5)

Beans and Greens Soup©‡†

>   2 cups cooked white beans
>   2 tablespoons olive oil
>   2 medium cloves garlic, crushed
>   1 large onion, chopped
>   1 bay leaf
>   1 stalk celery, diced
>   2 medium carrots, diced
>   1 teaspoon salt
>   Fresh black pepper, to taste
>   6 cups water or bone broth or vegetable or chicken broth
>   ½ lb. fresh chopped escarole, spinach, chard, or collards
>   (or a combination)

In a 4- to 6-quart soup pot, sauté the onions and garlic in olive oil over low heat. When onions are soft, add bay leaf, celery, carrot, salt, and pepper. Stir and sauté another 5 minutes. Add broth or water and cover. Simmer about 20 minutes. Add cooked beans and your choice of greens. Cover and continue to simmer, over very low heat, another 15 to 20 minutes. Serve immediately or refrigerate and reheat. (Serves 4 to 5)

Black Bean Stew©‡

> 1 tablespoon olive oil
> 1 large onion, diced
> 2 medium cloves garlic, minced
> 2 medium sweet potatoes or yams, peeled and diced
> 1 medium bell pepper, diced
> 14½ oz. can diced tomatoes or 2 cups fresh plum tomatoes, diced
> ½ cup water
> 1 small hot green chili pepper
> Two 16-oz. cans black beans, drained and rinsed or 3 to 4 cups
>   home-cooked black beans
> 1 ripe mango, peeled, pitted, and diced or rehydrated dried mango
> 1 ripe banana cut into ½-inch slices
> ½ cup chopped fresh cilantro
> ½ teaspoon sea salt

In large soup pot, heat oil over medium heat and add onion. Cook until softened, about 4 minutes. Stir in garlic and cook another 3 minutes. Stir in yam, bell pepper, tomatoes, chili, and water; bring to a boil. Reduce heat to low, cover, and simmer until yams are tender but not soft, 10 to 15 minutes. Stir in beans and simmer gently, uncovered, until heated through, about 5 minutes. Stir in mango and banana and cook 1 minute more, until heated through. Stir in cilantro and salt. If desired, serve over steamed quinoa. (Serves 4 to 6)

VEGETABLE DISHES

Greens Skillet†‡§

This is a terrific source of dietary sulfur and antioxidants. The coconut oil is very healthy and has a great taste. Olive oil is also good. Avoid canola or corn oil.

> 2 tablespoons coconut oil, olive oil,
>   or bone broth
> 3 tablespoons bone broth
> ½ pound Yukon Gold potatoes, diced
> ½ pound fresh shiitake mushrooms, diced
> 1 red bell pepper, diced
> 1 small butternut squash, peeled and diced
> 1 shallot, finely chopped
> 1 or 3 garlic, minced
> Soy sauce or liquid amino acids to taste
> 2 cups chopped collards, kale, or other greens
> 4 sprigs fresh sage or rosemary

Place oil and broth in a large skillet over medium heat. Melt coconut oil (or olive oil or bone broth) and mix in potatoes, mushrooms, pepper, squash, garlic, and shallot. Season with soy sauce, salt, and pepper to taste. Cook 25 minutes, stirring occasionally, until potatoes are tender. Mix kale and herbs into skillet. Continue cooking 5 minutes until kale is wilted. Serve and enjoy!

Sautéed Greens†‡§

Gently cooking the greens helps cut the bitterness. A wonderful variation is the addition of roasted sweet potatoes or yams that are cut up and stirred into the greens just before serving.

> 1 pound kale, collards, or other greens sliced into ¼-inch strips
> 1½ tablespoons extra virgin olive oil or coconut oil
> 1 large shallot, peeled and sliced very thin
> 1 clove garlic, chopped fine
> 3 tablespoons bone broth
> Liquid amino acids or soy sauce to taste
> ¼ cup of sesame seeds
> Grate ½ inch of ginger
> ¼ teaspoon of red paper flakes
> ⅛ teaspoon algae
> 1 teaspoon dried kelp

Wash kale thoroughly and drain but do not dry. Heat a large skillet with bone broth and sauté the shallot and garlic for 2 minutes. Stir in ginger and greens. Cook until wilted (1 to 2 minutes). Add red pepper flakes and serve.

Coconut Creamed Greens†§

This is a terrific way to tame the bitterness of the dark leafy greens. Adding something with a higher fat content cuts the bitterness. Since most people with MS are trying to avoid dairy, use coconut milk or nut butter in the place of any recipes that call for cream. This recipe and the one following are excellent examples of doing just that.

 2 heads kale, collards, or other dark greens
 1 cup bone broth
 2 tablespoons coconut oil or olive oil
 1 cup coconut milk
 ½ inch of ginger root, grated
 ½ to 1 teaspoon dried turmeric
 ½ to 1 teaspoon ground coriander
 ½ to 1 teaspoon ground cumin
 ½ to 1 teaspoon dried kelp
 ¼ teaspoon sugar
 1 teaspoon dried kelp
 Salt and fresh ground white pepper, to taste

Slice greens into 1/4-inch strips; let rest for 10 minutes prior to cooking. Place spices and kale in a large skillet, add chicken stock and simmer over medium heat until skillet is almost dry, 10 minutes. Add the oil and cook, stirring, for 2 minutes. Add coconut milk and sugar, season with salt and white pepper, and cook for another 6 to 8 minutes.

Cabbage Instead of Rice†

Shred cabbage and serve instead of rice when cooking an Asian dish.

Creamed Turnips or Rutabaga†

Buy an organic rutabaga, peel, cut up, cook in a bit of water, mash, and add a quarter cup of unsweetened soy milk and small amount of powdered ginger. Stir and enjoy warm. Or freeze and eat later.

Almond Nut Butter Creamed Greens†

3 tablespoons bone broth
1 onion, sliced into rings
1 to 2 garlic cloves minced
8 cups greens sliced into 1/4-inch strips.
¼ cup bone broth
2 teaspoons miso or soy sauce
¼ cup almond butter or other nut butter of your choice
Dried kelp
Salt to taste

Slice onions/greens and let sit for 10 minutes prior to cooking. Sauté onions and garlic in the bone broth. Add greens and cook another 5 minutes. Place in blender with broth and pulse until smooth. Then add remaining ingredients and blend (add the almond butter last to keep the blades from jamming). Add salt to taste.

Steamed Asparagus and Red Peppers†‡

Asparagus and red peppers are both very rich in organic sulfur. My kids enjoy this a great deal, and so do I.

1 bunch asparagus
2 large red peppers
2 tablespoons Balsamic vinegar
3 tablespoons chicken broth

Wash and break asparagus (save the stems to put in the pot in which you boil bones or veggies for broth or make into a creamed green soup). Seed and slice the red peppers (save the seeds and extra pieces to put in the pot for broth). Put the broth in a skillet, cover. When the broth is simmering, add the asparagus and red peppers. Simmer for 3 minutes but not longer than 5 minutes; the vegetables should still be crisp, not wilted.

Optional: Add one minced garlic and 1 tablespoon of flax oil as a dressing.

Sweet Potatoes, Easy Microwave Methods‡

Select a sweet potato or yam. Poke with a fork several times. Cook in microwave 5 minutes, turn, and cook 5 more minutes, turn, and cook 5 more minutes. Peel and eat plain. Or add coconut oil, olive oil, or flax oil as a dressing.

Parsnips (or Carrots)‡

Buy unwaxed organic parsnips, peel, chop into finger-length sticks, and cook in cooking spray and a tiny bit of water until tender. Eat plain. No seasoning, sugar, or salt is needed.

Spiced Lentil Casserole©†

> 1½ cups lentils, well rinsed
> 2 tablespoons sesame oil
> 3 cloves garlic, crushed
> 1 stalk celery, chopped
> 1 large onion, chopped
> ½ teaspoon salt
> 1 cup shredded, unsweetened coconut
> ½ teaspoon cinnamon
> ½ teaspoon powdered ginger
> ½ teaspoon turmeric
> 2 large green apples, washed and diced

Simmer lentils, covered, in 2½ cups water for 30 to 40 minutes, until tender. While they are cooking, in a wok or heavy skillet, sauté remaining ingredients, except apples, in oil until tender. Add water as necessary. Add apples and cook 10 more minutes, covered. Combine with cooked lentils in a casserole dish. (Serves 4)

Chili Pie©

1 cup chopped onion
½ tablespoon coconut or olive oil
1–2 teaspoons chili powder
1 tsp. ground cumin
½ teaspoon garlic powder
¼ teaspoon salt
15-oz. can red kidney beans, well drained
1½ cups cooked brown rice
½ cup Brewer's yeast
1½ cups coconut or nut milk
½ cup ground flax seeds
+ ½ cup boiling water
Green pepper, onion rings,
        and salsa for garnish, optional

In a large saucepan, cook onion in oil until softened. Stir in chili powder, cumin, garlic powder, and salt, cooking 1 more minute. Stir in beans, rice, brewer's yeast, milk, and flax seed and water combination. Spread in a 10-inch pie plate and bake, uncovered, at 350 degrees for about 20 minutes or until center is just set. Allow to sit for 10 minutes before serving. Garnish with green pepper and onion rings and salsa, if desired. (Serves 6)

Broccoli and Mushrooms ©‡

    1 lb. extra-firm tofu
    2 tablespoons wheat-free tamari (low-sodium soy sauce)
    3 tablespoons olive oil, divided
    2 teaspoons peeled and minced fresh ginger
    2 cloves garlic, minced
    2 cups broccoli florets
    2 cups sliced mushrooms
    1 red bell pepper, cut into thin strips
    1 tablespoon arrowroot or cornstarch
    1 tablespoon dry sherry
    ½ teaspoon cayenne or ¼ teaspoon hot-pepper flakes
    1 teaspoon sesame oil

Slice tofu into cubes. Toss with tamari and set aside for 5 to 10 minutes. In a wok or large nonstick skillet, heat 1 tbs. oil over high heat. When oil is hot, lower heat to medium-high and add scallions, ginger, and garlic; stir-fry for 30 seconds. Drain tofu, reserving tamari, and add tofu, stir-frying for 2 more minutes. Remove from pan and set aside. Using a fork or small whisk, mix reserved tamari with arrowroot or cornstarch, sherry, and cayenne in a small bowl. Set aside. Heat another 1 tbs. oil in wok over high heat. Add broccoli, mushrooms, and bell pepper and stir-fry for 2 minutes. Add ¼ cup water and bring to boil. Cover wok and reduce heat to medium, steaming vegetables about 5 minutes until slightly tender. Return tofu to wok.

    Stir reserved tamari mixture into wok and cook over medium heat until thickened and thoroughly heated; do not overcook vegetables. Add sesame oil and salt and pepper to taste and adjust seasonings if you desire a spicier dish. Serve immediately or make ahead and refrigerate until ready to serve. Reheat carefully; flavors are enhanced when the dish sits overnight.

Roasted Veggies©‡

    1 each red and yellow bell pepper, cut into large chunks
    2 red or yellow onions, peeled and cut into thick wedges
    2 medium zucchini, trimmed and cut into medium chunks
    1 medium eggplant or 4 baby eggplants, trimmed and cut
        into chunks
    1 fennel bulb, thickly sliced (gives a licorice flavor)
    2 large tomatoes, quartered or 8 plum tomatoes, halved
    8 large cloves garlic, peeled
    2 tablespoon olive oil
    Fresh rosemary sprigs
    ¼ teaspoon salt and pepper, or to taste

In a single layer, spread peppers, onion, zucchini, eggplant, and fennel in lightly oiled shallow roasting pan (you may use any combination of vegetables you desire). Arrange tomato pieces and garlic cloves among the vegetables and brush all with olive oil. Place rosemary sprigs among vegetables and grind some pepper over top. Sprinkle salt over all. Roast at 425 degrees for 20 to 30 minutes, turning vegetables after 15 minutes. Serve immediately or allow to cool and serve at room temperature. Leftovers will enhance a salad or side dish. (Serves 6)

Nutty Green Rice©

 1 cup brown basmati rice
 2 cups water
 ¼ to ½ teaspoon salt
 ½ cup almonds
 1 bunch parsley
 1 clove garlic
 1½ tablespoons lemon juice
 1½ tablespoons olive oil
 ½ cucumber, diced
 Pepper to taste

Bring water to a boil, add rice and salt, stir, and simmer, covered, for 45 minutes. Remove from heat and let sit for another 10 minutes; remove cover and allow to cool. While rice is cooking, blend almonds, parsley, garlic, and oil in a food processor. When rice is cool, stir with nut mixture and add pepper to taste. Garnish with cucumber if desired. (Serves 4)

Brown Rice and Peas©

Add 1 cup of green peas (either fresh and lightly steamed or frozen and just defrosted baby peas) to 2 cups of cooked brown rice. Top with your favorite herbs and flax oil to taste. (Serves 4)

Pasta and Beans©

16-oz. can white beans (pea, navy, great northern)
1–3 tablespoons olive oil
1 large onion, chopped
2 carrots, chopped
2 tablespoon dried basil or 1/4 cup chopped fresh basil
1 teaspoon dried oregano
16-oz. can tomatoes or 4 tomatoes, peeled, seeded, and chopped
½ cup bean liquid
1–2 teaspoon salt
½ lb. rice elbow gluten-free macaroni

Drain beans, reserving liquid. Heat olive oil in a heavy casserole dish. Add onions, carrots, oregano, and basil and cook until vegetables are wilted. Add tomatoes, bean liquid, salt, and pepper. Cover and simmer for about 10 minutes, until the vegetables are tender. Add the drained beans and simmer for another 20 minutes. Meanwhile, cook and drain the macaroni. Toss with olive oil and then mix with the bean sauce. (Serves 4)

NON-VEGETARIAN DISHES

Green Tea Pot Roast*‡

Grass-fed meat will be more tender and the nutrition will be more available to your body. If you have difficulty finding loose green tea, you can try an organic food store or search the Internet. Roast the meat slowly, preferably at 180 to 225 degrees. Keep the meat medium rare.

> 2 to 3 tablespoons loose green tea or 3 to 4 bags of green tea
> 2 pounds of pork, beef, or bison roast

Use leaf green tea to coat your roast. The phytonutrients, all of the great antioxidants in tea, will seep into the meat and tenderize it nicely. My family loves to have all of our roasts covered with a thick coating of green tea. They love how tender the meat is and how great it tastes. I love that they are getting another great source of antioxidants, too.

Rice Pasta Primavera with Chicken©

    2 cups uncooked rice pasta (noodles, spaghetti, elbows)
    1 large whole chicken breast, cut into strips
    1 each: red, yellow, green bell pepper cut in thin strips
    3–4 scallions, chopped
    2 cloves garlic, minced
    1 tablespoon olive or coconut oil
    ¼ cup fresh basil, finely chopped
    1 teaspoon paprika
    1 cup chicken broth
    3 tablespoon balsamic vinegar
    ½ cup black olives, halved (optional)

Cook rice pasta according to package directions. While pasta is cooking, in wok or heavy frying pan, stir-fry chicken strips, garlic, scallions, basil, and paprika in oil for about 5 minutes; add peppers and cook for 3 minutes. Add chicken broth and cook a few more minutes, until veggies have the desired texture. Remove from heat and add vinegar. Spoon over drained rice pasta and garnish with optional olives and extra olive oil as needed. (Serves 4)

Chicken Cutlets with Grape-Shallot Sauce‡

This quick sauté pairs wine and grapes in a luscious sauce. If you've never used grapes in a sauce before, try it — you won't be disappointed. This is simple enough for a weeknight, but elegant enough for entertaining. Serve with mashed sweet potatoes.

¼ cup non-gluten containing flour
4 chicken breast cutlets, trimmed of fat (about 1 pound)
1 teaspoon kosher salt
¼ teaspoon freshly ground pepper
5 teaspoon olive oil
1 cup thinly sliced shallots
2 cups halved seedless green, red, or black grapes
1 cup white wine
1 cup bone broth
2 tablespoons chopped fresh parsley

Place flour in a shallow dish. Sprinkle chicken with salt and pepper. Dredge the chicken in the flour (reserve excess flour). Heat 3 teaspoons oil in a large skillet over medium-high heat. Cook the chicken until golden on the first side, 2 to 4 minutes. Reduce heat to medium, turn the chicken, and cook until the other side is golden, 2 to 4 minutes more. Transfer to a plate.

Add the remaining 2 teaspoons oil to the pan and heat over medium heat. Add shallots and cook, stirring, until just starting to brown, 2 to 3 minutes. Add grapes and cook, stirring occasionally, until just starting to brown, 2 to 3 minutes. Sprinkle with 5 teaspoons of the reserved flour and stir. Add wine and broth; bring to a boil, stirring constantly. Reduce heat to a simmer and cook, stirring occasionally and scraping up any browned bits, until the sauce is reduced and thickened, about 8 minutes. Stir in parsley.

Return the chicken to the pan, turning to coat with sauce, and cook until heated through, about 2 minutes. Serve the chicken with the sauce on top.

Quinoa, Mexican Style©‡

½ lb. onions, chopped
1 teaspoon minced garlic
½ tablespoon olive oil
1 cup quinoa
1 cup chicken stock
1 cup drained, canned Italian plum tomatoes
1 cup tomato juice from canned tomatoes
½ to 1 whole jalapeno or serrano chili, seeded and chopped
2 tablespoons chopped fresh cilantro

Sauté the onion and garlic in hot oil in a heavy-bottom pot large enough to hold remaining ingredients. When onion is soft, add quinoa, chicken stock, plum tomatoes, tomato juice, and chili. Bring to boil; reduce heat, cover, and cook for about 10 minutes, until quinoa is tender. Sprinkle the coriander over quinoa mixture and serve. (Serves 6 as a side dish)

Turkey Loaf©‡

½ cup ground flax seed + ½ cup boiling water
¼ cup mushrooms, sautéed
½ cup shredded carrot
¼ cup orange juice
¼ cup whole oats*
2 tablespoons parsley
Salt and pepper
¼ teaspoon poultry seasoning
1 lb. ground turkey

Mix ingredients, shape into loaf, and place in 9-inch pie plate. Bake at 350 degrees for 35 minutes. Serve immediately. (Serves 4–5)
　　*There is controversy concerning the gluten-free status of oats; do not use this recipe if you are concerned that you may have a reaction.

Turkey Stroganoff Skillet©

1 lb. ground turkey
12 oz. can vegetable juice or tomatoe juice, low sodium preferable
10 oz. chicken broth
¾ cup water
½ cup mushrooms, sautéed
2 teaspoons minced onion
1 teaspoon dried parsley
1 teaspoon Worcestershire sauce
½ teaspoon thyme
⅛ teaspoon pepper
¼ lb. rice noodles (any shape)

In a large skillet, brown turkey. Stir in remaining ingredients. Bring to boil; cover and simmer 15 minutes. (Serves 6)

Baked Turkey or Chicken Stew©

2 stalks celery, thinly sliced
1 medium red or green pepper, chopped
1 medium onion, chopped
1 clove garlic, minced
2 tablespoons olive oil
4 teaspoons rice or flour
1 tablespoon chili powder
½ teaspoon dried thyme, crushed
½ teaspoon dried rosemary, crushed
⅛ teaspoon ground red pepper
14½ oz. can stewed tomatoes
12 oz. can V-8 juice
1½ cups chopped cooked turkey or chicken (good use for leftovers)

Sauté celery, pepper, onion, and garlic in olive oil until tender. Stir in remaining ingredients, except for turkey or chicken. Cook and stir until bubbly. Add turkey or chicken. Transfer to 1½-quart casserole. Cover; bake at 375 degrees for 15–20 minutes or until heated through. Season with salt and pepper. Serve over cooked brown rice. (Serves 4)

Fish Creole©

    1-2 tablespoons coconut olive oil
    1 onion, chopped
    ½ cup thinly sliced celery
    1 chopped green pepper
    1 clove garlic, minced
    2 tablespoons fresh parsley or 2 teaspoons dried
    1 bay leaf
    ¼ teaspoons rosemary, crumbled
    28 oz. can tomatoes with liquid
    1 lb. fish fillets, cut into bite-size pieces
    2 cups cooked brown rice

Heat oil in a large saucepan and lightly sauté the onion, celery, pepper, and garlic until soft. Add parsley, rosemary, and tomatoes. Simmer, uncovered, about 20 minutes. Add fish fillets in small pieces and simmer until cooked through, about 5–10 minutes more. Remove bay leaf. Serve over hot cooked rice with a green salad. (Serves 4)

Lamb-Zucchini Casserole©†

1 lb. boneless lamb
1 cup chopped onion
1 clove garlic, minced
Two 10-oz. packages frozen spinach, thawed and well drained
1 teaspoon dried basil
Dash nutmeg
⅔ cup chicken or vegetable broth
1 teaspoon cornstarch
2 small zucchini, thinly sliced
¼ cup Brewer's yeast

In a large skillet, brown lamb, onion, and garlic. Drain fat. In a bowl, combine spinach, ½ teaspoon basil, and nutmeg and add to meat, mixing well. Stir in mozzarella. In a separate bowl, combine broth and cornstarch and mix well. Add to lamb mixture and spread all in a casserole dish, approximately 10 inches by 6 inches. Arrange zucchini slices on top and sprinkle with Brewer's yeast and remaining basil. Bake covered at 350 degrees for 30 minutes. Uncover and bake 5–10 minutes more. Allow to sit for 5 minutes before serving. (Serves 6–8)

Pineapple Salmon©*

2 cups unsweetened pineapple juice
4 teaspoons wheat-free tamari
        (low-sodium soy sauce)
Four 5–6-oz. salmon steaks

In a small saucepan, bring pineapple juice to a boil; lower heat to medium and cook until juice is reduced to 1 cup. Transfer to a small bowl and allow to cool. Mix in soy sauce. Place salmon in shallow casserole dish and pour the pineapple marinade over, turning occasionally. Allow to sit for 2 hours. Remove from marinade and sauté salmon in a large nonstick skillet over medium-high heat for about 5 minutes on each side, being careful not to overcook. While salmon is cooking, cook remaining marinade in small saucepan over medium-low heat for about 5 more minutes, until it is again reduced by half. Brush top of each salmon steak with marinade and serve immediately. (Serves 4)

DESSERTS

Aronia Fruit Salad‡

Mix together:

> 1 cup Aronia berries – chopped finely or put through food processor
> 1 cut-up apple
> 1 cup-up orange
> 1 cup chopped grapes
> ½ cup chopped nuts of your choice
> 1 teaspoon cinnamon (decreases the amount of sugar you will need)
> 2 tablespoons honey
> 2 tablespoons other sweetener, or to taste needed

Fruit Pudding‡

This is as pleasant pudding that is free of both dairy and eggs. One could substitute any type of berries in place of the Aronia berries.

> 1 cup Aronia berries (or cranberries)
> 1 cup of cherries
> 2 cups grape juice, or other deep-red or purple juice
> 1-2 tablespoons honey or ½ cup sugar (to taste)
> 1 teaspoon cinnamon
> ½ teaspoon nutmeg
> ⅓ cup Tapioca (minute or pearl)

Bring to boil and cook five minutes, stirring continuously. Cool; may also be served warm.

Sweet Potato Squash Delight

    1 medium butternut squash, peeled and cut into chunks
    2–3 medium sweet potatoes, peeled and cut into chunks
    1/2 teaspoon ginger
    1 teaspoon cinnamon
    Dash nutmeg
    1/4 –1/2 cup almond, oat, coconut, or rice milk
        (add enough to make creamy)
    Sliced or slivered almonds

Steam squash and sweet potatoes until tender. When cool enough to handle, puree in food processer. While continuing to process, add ginger, cinnamon, nutmeg, and milk. Put in 1 1/2-quart casserole and sprinkle with sliced or slivered almonds. Bake at 350 degrees for about 15 minutes. (Serves 10)
    Note: If preparing ahead, do not bake until just before serving.

Squash Pudding or Pie‡

I was missing pumpkin pie and so was my family. I came up with this option, which they said was fabulous. I use a VitaMix machine to grind up the squash seeds to make part of the milk that goes into the pie. If you don't have a VitaMix, substitute with ground flax seeds.

All the seeds from a baked squash or 1 cup freshly ground flax seed
2 cups cooked orange squash, pumpkin, yam, or sweet potatoes
½ cup flax seed
¼ cup hemp seed
4 tablespoons of minute tapioca (or tapioca flour)
2 cups of non-dairy milk of choice
2 teaspoons cinnamon
½ teaspoon cloves
¼ teaspoon nutmeg
¼ allspice
2-5 Tablespoons of honey or natural maple syrup
coconut oil, to grease pan

Grind the flax seed in a coffee-grinder. Mix with 2 tablespoons boiling water and let sit. If the hemp seed isn't already cracked, grind the hemp seeds. Dump the cooked squash, squash seeds, spices, and the liquid ingredients (including the flax seed and boiling water combination) into the VitaMix. Start on low, turn dial to high and then mix on high until thoroughly mixed and the squash seeds thoroughly pulverized (about 4 minutes). Add the sweetener and tapioca. Check the taste and adjust accordingly. Bring to boil on the stove and simmer for five minutes. If you are making a pudding you may let cool, and serve. On the other hand, if you wish to serve as a pie rather than a pudding do the following.

Grease a pan with coconut oil and pour in the squash mixture into the greased pan. Bake in a 350 degree oven until a knife inserted into the pie comes out clean (approximately 45 minutes).

Banana Custard Pie©

    ½ cup hot water
    1 tablespoon gelatin powder (1 envelope)
    ½ cup pineapple juice
    2 tablespoon coconut oil (or 1 tablespoon flax meal + 2 tablespoons
        boiling water)
    ¼ cup coconut oil
    ½ teaspoon vanilla
    4 bananas, cut into pieces
    2 tablespoon unsweetened coconut

Combine hot water and gelatin in blender until gelatin is completely dis-solved. With the blender running, add pineapple juice, flax meal water, oil, vanilla, and 3 bananas. Slice another banana into a pie dish or other glass dish. Sprinkle with coconut. Pour blender mixture over banana slices and garnish with more coconut. (Serves 6)

Rice Pudding©

    1 cup uncooked short-grain brown rice
    1¼ cups coconut milk
    1¼ cups water
    ½ teaspoon salt
    1 tablespoon brown rice syrup or honey
    1 teaspoon cinnamon
    Chopped almonds, sunflower seeds,
        or other nuts of choice (optional)

Combine water and coconut milk in heavy pot; bring to boil, adding rice and salt. Simmer, covered (do not stir) for about 45 minutes or more, until liquid is mostly absorbed and rice is soft. Remove from heat and allow to cool for 15 minutes. Stir in brown rice syrup and cinnamon and top with nuts or seeds as desired. Can be used for dessert or breakfast. (Serves 4)

Berry Freeze©‡

> 1 lb. frozen strawberries, slightly thawed, or
>   1 pint fresh berries, frozen slightly
> ½ cup soy, hemp, or almond milk
> ¼ cup tofu
> 3 tablespoons all-fruit strawberry jam
> Fresh strawberries for garnish (optional)

Blend slightly frozen berries in food processor. Slowly add ricotta and then jam, blending all the while. Serve immediately, garnished with a fresh strawberry, if desired. (Serves 4)

Poached Peaches with Strawberry Sauce©‡

> 6-oz. can frozen unsweetened apple juice concentrate, thawed
> 1 cup water
> 1 tablespoon finely grated lemon peel
> 1 teaspoon vanilla extract
> 4 medium ripe peaches or nectarines (pears are a winter alternative)
> 4 sprigs fresh mint for garnish (optional)
> 2 cups fresh strawberries, hulled and washed
> ¼ cup orange juice (unsweetened)
> Pinch each of ground cinnamon and nutmeg

For sauce, combine strawberries, orange juice, cinnamon, and nutmeg in blender or food processor. Process until smooth. Sauce is excellent for any poached fruit.

For peaches, in a medium saucepan, mix apple juice, water, lemon peel, and vanilla; bring to boil and reduce heat. Cover and simmer for 10 minutes. Add peaches (or other desired fruit) and poach, partially covered over low heat, for 7 to 8 minutes. Remove from heat and allow to cool in liquid. When cool, carefully slip skins off peaches, cut in half lengthwise, and remove pits. Spoon strawberry sauce into 4 dessert plates, making a little pool. On each plate, arrange 2 peach halves in the center and garnish with mint. (Serves 4)

Baked Apples©‡

⅓ cup golden raisins
2 tablespoons apple juice
6 cooking apples, cored
1½ cups water
¼ cup frozen unsweetened apple juice concentrate
2 teaspoons pure vanilla extract
1 teaspoon cinnamon
1 teaspoon arrowroot

Remove peel from top third of each apple and arrange in a small baking dish. In a medium saucepan, combine with other ingredients and bring to a boil, stirring frequently. Reduce heat and simmer 2–3 minutes, until slightly thickened. Distribute raisins, filling centers of each apple. Pour sauce over apples and bake, uncovered, at 350 degrees for 1 to 1½ hours. Baste occasionally and remove from oven when apples are pierced easily with a fork. Spoon juice over apples and serve warm. (Serves 6)

Baked Apples with Cashew Topping©

4 firm cooking apples
½ cup raisins or currants
½ cup raw cashew pieces
Vanilla extract and cinnamon

Cut apples horizontally through peel around the middle to keep from splitting during baking. Core apples and fill centers with 2 tablespoon raisins each. Sprinkle with cinnamon. Bake at 350 degrees for 45 minutes or until tender. While apples are baking, blend cashews in blender, adding water gradually until the consistency is smooth. Add a few drops of vanilla extract and cover each warm apple with cashew topping. (Serves 4)

Sautéed Apples©

Use this as topping for pancakes, waffles, or French toast.

> 2 apples
> ½ tablespoon coconut oil
> 2 teaspoons cinnamon
> 2-3 tablespoons apple juice

Thinly slice washed apples and sauté in coconut oil and cinnamon until softened. Add apple juice and simmer uncovered for a few more minutes, stirring.

Banana-Strawberry-Orange Cream©

> 1 cup strawberries
> 2 medium bananas
> 1 cup orange juice
> 1 medium apple
> ¼ cup raw cashew pieces
> Lemon juice (optional)

Wash and hull strawberries; peel and slice bananas. (Bananas may be tossed in lemon juice to preserve color.) Combine orange juice, cored apple, and cashew pieces in a blender; blend and pour over strawberries and bananas. (Serves 3)

Super Detox Smoothies and Teas©

Smoothies

Smoothies can be a great complement to dietary program and help make "food as medicine" delicious and nutritious.

Brew one quart of strong tea. Let the tea steep 10-15 minutes. Store it in the refrigerator.

> Green tea
> Nettle tea (try Traditional Medicinals)
> Licorice tea
> Tulsi tea (try Organic India)
> Detox tea

Use 4-6 oz. of the above for your base liquid for your smoothie. Place it in a blender.

Add 2-4 oz. of:

> Chilled pomegranate juice
> Welch's unsweetened purple grape juice
> Acai juice
> "Morning blend" or any Knudsen Organic
> "just" juice
> Add ½ cup of frozen blueberries, blackberries, or raspberries
>   (preferably organic).

Add one to two tablespoons of ground flax seed (e.g., Bob's Red Mill Ground Flax Meal). Store extra ground flax seed in fridge. It will keep for 3-4 weeks.

Add any sweet whole fruit of your choice. For example, pineapple, banana, peach, in-season melon, ripe pear, ripe (sweet) mango, or unsweetened organic applesauce. Avoid processed fruit containing high-fructose corn syrup.

Protein and additional nutrients:

Protein drink (add two tablespoons):
  Rice protein powder
  Soy powder
  Whole oats soaked overnight in the refrigerator in soy, almond, rice, or dairy milk
  One scoop or tablespoon instant greens
  ¼ to 1 teaspoon spirulina, chlorella, or blue-green algae
  Add ¼ cup of crushed ice if you like your smoothie cold.

Spices to cut the bitterness – any combination of the following lesson the bitterness and can further boost the health benefit of the detox.

Cinnamon:	1-2 teaspoons
Cloves:	¼ teaspoon
Cardamom:	¼ teaspoon
Nutmeg:	¼ teaspoon
Organic cocoa:	1 teaspoon

Blend until it is of the right consistency for you. You may need to add more tea if it seems too thick to you.

Detox Tea

Base Detox Tea can be made from different herb tea combinations, either from tea bags or home brewed from bulk herb. Simmer in two quarts of hot water for 10-15 minutes, then cover and turn off the stove and allow it to cool 20 minutes or so. Strain and discard the loose tea. Store in the refrigerator. This stays good for a week to ten days. Use the herb tea mixes above or any combination of those below:

> 4 tablespoons of loose green tea
> 2 tablespoons of lemon balm leaf
> 2 tablespoons of dried hawthorne
> 2 tablespoons of dried elder berries
> 1 tablespoon of fresh rosemary chopped
> 1 teaspoon of fresh ground turmeric
> 1 half teaspoon of fresh ground cinnamon
> 1 tablespoon ground milk thistle

Chapter Nine
THE SYNERGY BETWEEN NEURO-MUSCULAR ELECTRICAL STIMULATION AND NUTRITION

Multiple sclerosis (MS) affects more than 400,000 Americans. The majority diagnosed with relapsing remitting MS will transition to secondary progressive MS within 15 years of the initial diagnosis.[281] Within 25 years, 85 percent of relapsing, remitting MS patients transition into the secondary progressive phase of MS. Once people transition to a secondary progressive phase of MS, they will slowly, progressively deteriorate. Treatment goals are to stabilize the patient and slow the deterioration, since there is no reliable method to return people to full function again.

Although MS is believed to be an autoimmune disease with antibodies being generated to attack and destroy myelin, which is the lining around nerve cells, we do not know what causes the body to begin making those antibodies. Nor do we understand what causes the transition from relapsing remitting MS to secondary progressive MS. It is also not clear why, in spite of the absence of acute flares causing muscular weakness in secondary progressive MS, patients experience a relentless loss of strength and endurance. MRI findings do not change, other than to show gradual reduction in brain and spinal-cord volume over time. The presumption is that brain cells are dying. The scientific term is *neurodegeneration*, and it has been the presumed cause of the accumulating disability and loss of function in both secondary and progressive MS.[281,282]

Few treatments are available that have been shown to effectively halt the progression or restore lost functional capacities. Potent drugs have been used to suppress the white blood cells so they cannot make the antibodies into myelin. Bone marrow transplants have not been very helpful. Some cancer chemotherapy drugs, such as mitoxantrone, have slowed the rate of progression.[283-286]

Rehabilitation to maximize function as the patient loses strength and function is the main focus of treatment during the progressive phase of MS. Physical exercise in the form of yoga, weight training, Pilates, and physical therapy have all been shown to be helpful in improving the quality of life as patients experience decline.[287,288]

Fatigue is the most frequent severely disabling problem for MS patients. Fatigue worsens over time and becomes progressively more disabling for most MS patients, leading to ever-decreasing amounts of physical activity. Stimulants like Provigil and Ritalin are prescribed with only modest benefit. Patients are encouraged to maintain a limited workout program to maintain strength, without causing worsening fatigue from having exercised. It can be a fine line for many patients between how much exercise they can do and still go to work and maintain family responsibilities.

Electrical therapy has been around for many years, and has been used in MS to treat pain since the 1970s in the form of transcutaneous electrical stimulation, also called TENS. In TENS, low doses of electrical current are applied through patches placed on the skin. It helps deplete the messenger signals for pain and can decrease the severity of nerve-related pain in MS.

Other methods of using electricity to improve muscle strength have since been developed. Electrical therapy has more recently been used to aid in the development of muscle strength and prevent atrophy of muscles. This form of electrical therapy, neuromuscular electrical stimulation (NMES), has been used primarily in athletes to speed recovery from orthopedic injuries. A few studies have been done in non-athletes with clinical applications. It has been used to prevent and treat musculoskeletal deterioration occurring after strokes, and has shown faster and more effective recovery, if NMES is used during rehabilitation after a stroke.[289] It has also been helpful in improving control of and decreasing spasms in patients with cerebral palsy and those with spinal cord injury.[290]

There is also another type of electrical stimulation called functional electrical stimulation (FES). In this type of stimulation, an electrical impulse is sent to the nerve that goes to the muscles in the leg at knee level. It has been used to mimic cycling for thirty minutes and decrease foot drop. In both of these types of studies, decreased spasticity and improved endurance was noted.[291]

Bladder control clinics also use electrical stimulation to improve the strength of the bladder- and colon-sphincter muscles, with the intent to decrease bowel or bladder accidents. Incontinence, which is uncontrolled leakage of either urine or stool, is a major problem for many individuals with spinal cord injuries. McClurg[292] compared biofeedback and pelvic exercises coupled with either sham NMES or actual NMES. He found that the incontinence was reduced by eighty-five percent in the group using NMES-augmented pelvic exercise and biofeedback, compared to forty-seven percent in the group not using NMES augmentation. NMES treatments to improve bladder and bowel control appears to be promising and may be an area to discuss with your provider if you are having problems with incontinence related to MS.

Although no other cases have been reported that used NMES in the setting of multiple sclerosis, the fact that NMES and FES have been helpful in so many clinical settings, including with neurological disorders, implies that it is likely to help more people than just me. This may be a useful and relatively safe way to help rehabilitate those with MS-related gait or fatigue disability.

At the University of Iowa, Dr. Rich Shields studies the use of NMES in individuals who were paralyzed due to a traumatic injury. I review twenty or more research studies each month as a member of the institutional review board that oversees research conducted on human subjects at the University of Iowa and the Iowa City VA. I had the good fortune to be assigned to review Rich Shields' study, so I learned about NMES and began to think it might help someone with MS. As a result of reviewing that study, I was inspired to request a trial of NMES for myself, which became very helpful in slowly rebuilding my muscle strength and endurance. Although NMES is not an FDA-approved treatment modality for multiple sclerosis, NMES does have FDA approval for the treatment of muscle spasm, muscle pain, and disuse atrophy, all of which are commonly seen in the setting of multiple sclerosis-related gait disability. Thus, if one works with their physician to document the presence of muscle spasm, muscle pain, and/or disuse atrophy, it would be much easier to get access to NMES to support rehabilitation of their gait using NMES and progressive exercise.

I used NMES in conjunction with a home exercise program that was supervised by a physical therapist who had experience using NMES to re-habilitate athletes. It was a slow process, requiring many hours of electrical stimulation each day. I used NMES during my daily home-exercise program to strengthen my lower back, and also during the day while doing usual my activities. The device I used was a 300 PV manufactured by EMPI. It was a small portable device that used rechargeable AA batteries.

Over the course of a year, I went from being dependent on a motor-ized scooter, to requiring one-to-two canes to walk, to being able to walk throughout the hospital and bicycle eighteen miles without any assistance. The potential mechanisms by which NMES results in functional gains are likely due to changes within the central nervous system (CNS), as well as within the muscle. Many experts have documented changes in the brain in response to exercise. These include more nerve growth factor (NGF), brain-derived neurotrophic growth factor (BDNF), insulin-like growth factor (ILGF), and glial growth factor (GGF), as well as a healthier immune function.[293-295] Transcutaneous electrical stimulation results in increased beta endorphins and reduced levels of inflammatory cytokines,[296] both of which have been demonstrated to be abnormal in people with progressive MS.[297] It is possible that NMES-augmented exercise results in favorable in-creases in multiple brain growth factors and down regulation of inflamma-tory molecules within the CNS, all of which should be helpful in the setting of secondary progressive MS.

The prime role of nutrition in the progression or remission of MS symp-toms has not been fully clarified by researchers. However, a number of studies have suggested that dietary factors may influence disease severity and or progression, particularly omega-3 fatty acids,[298-303] vitamin D,[304-308] and vitamin B_{12}[309].

Another area where nutrition may play a role is food allergies or sensi-tivities. Some experts have found an association of neurological symptoms with celiac disease,[310,311] while others have not.[312-314] If you think food sen-sitivities or allergies may be affecting you, keep a log of the food you eat each day. In addition, rate your pain, energy level, and other symptoms. Using a food-symptom diary can be very helpful in sorting out the possible links between food sensitivities and symptoms.

Problems with mitochondria, also called oxidative stress, have been im-plicated as a contributor to the loss of brain cells. In animal models of diseases such as Parkinson's, Alzheimer's, Huntington's, Amyotrophic Lat-eral Sclerosis (ALS), cerebral ischemia, and optic neuritis, mitochondrial dysfunction has been implicated as a contributing factor.[288,315-322] Reducing oxidative stress has been shown to protect brain cells in optic neuritis in experiments,[323] supporting the importance of reducing oxidative stress and nutrition in MS patients.

Another problem that can kill brain cells is something called excito-toxicity. Imagine a cell that is being driven so hard by excess ATP to respond, that it collapses from exhaustion. The cellular functions begin to deteriorate and more toxins form. The mitochondria, which are supposed to neutralize the toxins, become less and less effective. If the stimulation continues to drive the cell when it has no energy, the toxins build up and the mitochondria sends a message to the nucleus that it is time to die.

Studies have shown that brain-cell loss in MS is, in fact, mediated in part by excito-toxicity, oxidative stress, and damage to cellular mitochondria and cellular DNA.[324,325] Multiple experts have observed nutritional supplements and dietary interventions aimed at reducing oxidative stress to treat or prevent autoimmune diseases, including multiple sclerosis.[326-331]

Nutritional interventions targeting mitochondria with multiple simultaneous micronutrient support have not been studied in patients with multiple sclerosis. Science prefers to study one intervention at a time, so it knows what to attribute the beneficial or adverse response. It is too messy to analyze multiple interventions at once. Science would not have approved of an intervention that added the number of supplements that I did when I changed my nutritional focus. That means that I do not know, specifically, which micronutrients were most critical and which were not.

Subjectively, the addition of the intensive micronutrient support through the dietary changes and the supplements was associated with significant increase in the rate of my recovery. Furthermore, I observed that if I missed either NMES or my usual diet, I felt noticeably different within twenty-four hours. My energy seemed reduced, and my concentration not as clear. I believe they were synergistic in helping me improve.

I do not know the molecular changes that were occurring, but I can offer some theories about what was happening in my brain, spinal cord, and muscles with the electricity and nutrition that was likely synergistic in my case. I will review some very basic neuro-biology first.

Our brain cells connect to each other through little arms called dendrites and axons. It is likely, given what the literature says about exercise and the brain, that my additional exercise and/or NMES caused my brain to make more neuro-trophins, or brain cell growth factors, and the brain cells then received signals to grow more dendrites and axons. That requires energy in the form of ATP and omega-3 fatty acids to build the myelin insulation around the new connections. It makes sense that improving how the mitochondria generate ATP molecules (energy) is synergistic with exercise. It is like adding an extra engine to your car. You have more energy and more stamina.

The rate by which the brain cells respond to these messengers is likely therefore to be dependent, at least in part, on the availability of ATP generated in the mitochondria. A diet containing more B vitamins (particularly riboflavin and niacinamide) coupled with more ubiquinone, or coenzyme Q, should make it easier for mitochondria to make ATP and get rid of the toxins generated in the cells. That decreases the oxidative stress and makes for healthier mitochondria. If the mitochondria are healthier, the brain cells are healthier, and healthier brains are better able to respond to brain-growth factors formed in response to the higher level of physical activity.

Multiple studies have shown that excito-toxicity causes part of the damage in MS.[332-334] Excessive glutamate is present in the brain in the animal model of MS, experimental autoimmune encephalitis, and also in patients with an acute MS relapse, primary progressive MS, and secondary progressive MS.[335-337] The neurotransmitter most often involved with excito-toxicity in MS is glutamate. When glutamate becomes excessive, it can lead to too much calcium coming into the brain cell. The extra calcium can eventually kill the brain cell. But there are things one can do to moderate the effect of the extra glutamate.

There are things in our diet that can increase the amount of glutamate that we have in our brains. In some people, MSG (monosodium glutamate) and aspartame (NutraSweet®) cause increases in glutamate, which in turn causes excito-toxicity and neurological symptoms like headache, fatigue, and unexplained, vague neurological symptoms.

Because glutamate is involved in learning, it is important that our brain cells have glutamate; it is an excess of the substance that is the problem. The counterbalance to glutamate is a neurotransmitter called gamma amino butyric acid, or GABA. Because GABA cannot cross the blood-brain barrier, it must be made in the brain by sulfur-containing amino acids, like cysteine, taurine, and methionine. In fact, in studies of MS using mice, blocking glutamate synthesis with taurine or N-acetyl cysteine led to an increased amount of brain GABA and has reversed disability in mice.[338] I used N-acetyl cysteine, taurine, and nutrition to support the generation of glutathione, as strategies to help my brain make more GABA.

There are several case reports by Dr. Sandyk of secondary progressive multiple sclerosis in which regression of disability is documented.[339-354] In all cases, pulsed electro-magnet therapy was used, which gradually allowed the patients to recover some degree of function. Because magnetic and electrical fields have some similarities, one can speculate that there may be a similar mechanism of action, in some capacity shared by magnetic fields and electricity.

I cannot specify which of the interventions I used, electrotherapy or nutrition, was the most effective, or what combinations are required to receive the greatest benefit. However, I believe it is likely that there is considerable synergy between a diet rich in micronutrients, antioxidants, low-dose lithium, and NMES-augmented exercise. Further study is needed and will take place, slowly, step by step.

I have a wish list of the additional questions I'd love to see answered. Studies of the biochemical impact of NMES on brain growth factors, beta-endorphin, and inflammatory cytokines are needed. Additional basic-science studies of mitochondrial function, as well as the nutritional impact on mitochondrial function in patients with progressive multiple sclerosis, are needed. We do not yet have proof that what happened in me can be replicated in others. More study is needed.

I am currently working with my colleagues on a pilot study to investigate whether electrotherapy, combined with intensive nutrition, can help others with primary and secondary progressive MS. For any future studies of NMES, careful selection of study patients will be required to identify people who are willing and capable of complying with the intervention program. That is because there is substantial time commitment to complete the NMES sessions, there is discomfort without immediate benefit, and changes to the diet may be substantial.

Because NMES and a nutritional diet have a lower risk profile than most standard therapies (meaning the risk of negative side effects are few), it could be a very attractive option for patients with progressive MS, if my results can be replicated. Although many questions remain, I do believe my experience shows that greater recovery of function for people with progressive MS may be far more possible than has been appreciated. The hope of returning to walking may not have to be in vain for everyone who has gotten into a wheelchair because of progressive MS. NMES has been used in the setting of severe heart disease and lung disease safely. In those circumstances, a progressive exercise program was coupled with NMES over two to three months, leading to significant improvement in the quality of life scores.[355-361] Notably in those studies there were few problems with patient compliance or adverse events. In those studies, patients were severely disabled, much as patients with progressive MS are. It is likely, therefore, that the progressive MS patients might also experience improvements in the quality of life by coupling NMES and progressive exercise.

An excellent resource to guide both professionals and individuals who wish to utilize electrical stimulation of muscles can be found in the book *Application of Muscle/ Nerve Stimulation in Health and Disease,* published by Springer in 2008.[362] This brief monograph reviews the science behind the use of electrical stimulation, including a discussion of the changes in physiology and brain chemistry thay I discussed earlier. It then reviews the use of electrical therapy as a tool to restore motor function, including in the setting of neuromuscular diseases. The authors provide specific references and the parameters thay have been used to prevent muscle deterioration in patients following surgery, spinal cord injury, and bed rest, and note that electrical therapy is likely to be beneficial for those suffering from neurological and neuromuscular disorders. It is an excellent resource which can guide both the professional who oversees treatment with electrical stimulation and the patient.

Because the book provides a detailed chapter as a user's guide to the use of electrical stimulation for health, beauty, fitness, and rehabilitation, the book is an excellent resource for individuals who are using electrical stimulation on their own. In that chapter the authors provide a detailed review with specific instruction on the placement of electrodes and the specific parameters for electrical therapy. Having implanted electrical devices such as pacemakers, Baclofen pumps, and possibly heart disease and seizure disorders as well as serious poorly controlled diseases of any type would be contraindications for electrical therapy, meaning the use would not necessarily be safe.

While there is good evidence that muscle size and strength can be increased using electrical stimulation, improving actual coordination and function of the muscles requires willful contraction and exercise of the affected muscle groups. A physical therapist or other professional who understands exercise physiology is best equipped to analyze the person's current abilities and recommend the appropriate exercise programs to re-educate the muscles and improve their function. Thus, although an individual may be able to use electrical stimulation of muscles in their own home, guided by *Application of Muscle/ Nerve Stimulation in Health and Disease*, working with a professional who can design a home exercise program, will likely be much more successful at improving function and restoring a more normal gait pattern.

Again, while there is ample evidence suggesting electrical stimulation of muscles is generally well tolerated and may be beneficial to those with MS, there are no large research trials that have proven the safety or effectiveness of electrical therapy in maintaining muscle strength and stamina. As a result, anyone who pursues electrical stimulation of their muscles does so at their own risk. Talk to your physicians and therapists about electrical therapy to determine whether there are contraindications to a trial of electrical stimulation in your particular circumstances.

The risks of long-term electrical stimulation are not known. Some people with multiple sclerosis have problems with sensation on their skin. If they can't detect pain on their skin surface, they may accidently give themselves so much electrical current, that they give themselves an electrical burn on their skin. Although the public can purchase less-powerful electrical stimulation devices directly (i.e., no prescription from a doctor), I believe that it is critical to have a medical professional familiar with electrical therapy conduct the first use of the electrical stimulation device and establish initial treatment guidelines for anyone who wishes to use electrical stimulation for therapeutic reasons, for example, in the setting of a muscular or neurological disease like MS. Again, although neuromuscular electrical stimulation is not an FDA-approved modality for MS, it is approved for muscle spasm, muscle pain, and disuse atrophy, all of which are common in those who have gait disability due to their MS. Talk to your doctor about whether or not you have these diagnoses and request a referral to physical therapy to help control symptoms related to those problems. Look for a physical therapist with expertise using neuromuscular stimulation and request a test session. Then you can work with your therapist to see if you can get access to a device to use at home with a home exercise program.

Chapter Ten
FREQUENTLY ASKED QUESTIONS AND ANSWERS

I have often spoken publicly about my experience. In this section, I will provide answers to some of the common questions I have received that may not have been previously answered.

What do you do in your clinical practice?

I work in a Veterans Administration hospital as a physician, seeing patients with traumatic brain injuries and severe psychiatric disorders. I also see patients in primary care clinics who have common internal medicine problems. Usually I work with patients to fix their dietary choices first. I tell them that I am like a firefighter who has been called to cool off the inflammation in their bodies and their brains. I will do the best I can for them. I'll treat them to the best of my ability, but if they continue eating a high-carbohydrate diet with few fruits and vegetables they are spraying their body with gasoline. No matter how powerful my water hose, as long as they are stoking the fire with a high-carbohydrate diet, their disease will never cool off. I stress the importance of eating nine cups of fruits and vegetables every day before they eat grains or starchy vegetables.

I generally do not advocate the use of supplements until the individual has successfully implemented a diet that is rich in vegetables and fruits. I provide a list of specific nutrients and good food sources for those nutrients to teach people which foods they should be emphasizing in their diets. Once they have, depending on their personal and family health history, it may be appropriate to add specific supplements to improve specific aspects of the individual's biochemical functioning.

What did I do regarding my food consumption since I was initially diagnosed with MS?
In 2003, I began the Paleolithic diet. I eliminated grains, milk, and legumes. I continued to eat meat, poultry, fish, vegetables (including white potatoes), fruit, and eggs. By 2007, I had gone back to eating rice and, occasionally, beans.

In the summer of 2007, I took a blood test for food allergies, which identified marked sensitivity to eggs, pinto beans, and milk. I eliminated those from my diet in October. I started the four-day rotation diet, but did not maintain it. I was not keeping a food-symptom diary.

In November 2007, I started a neurostim program. At the end of December, I started an intensive diet, rich with a minimum of nine cups of fruits and vegetables a day. I ate four to six cups of cruciferous or onion family vegetables each day, and three cups of brightly colored vegetables or fruits. In January 2009, I went back to creating a food/symptom diary and began the elimination diet with the four-day rotation of foods. In March 2009, I eliminated all sources of cereal grasses to further restrict gluten exposure.

Why was I able to go from being dependant on a motorized scooter for four years, to return to walking, bicycling, and skiing?
Since I don't have a series of blood tests to identify how much my nutritional status changed, my inflammatory status, or any biological changes that were occurring, it is hard to say precisely what happened as I became stronger. I have several theories, which I'll share.

First – The neurostimulation that I started in November 2007, coupled with exercise, produced stronger, larger muscles and generated growth factors in the brain, which stimulates repair of myelin and grows new connections between brain cells. That prepared my brain to do repair work. The food made it possible for the brain cells to use the growth factors.

Second – I more vigorously eliminated the foods to which I had documented food sensitivity on the blood tests in the summer of 2007.

Third – I greatly increased the intake of B vitamins, co-enzyme Q, antioxidants, and organic sulfur with specific food choices. This resulted in a big boost of the micronutrients I was eating.

Fourth – I switched to eating entirely organic foods.

Fifth – I focused on eating food of every color each day.

Sixth – I eliminated white potatoes, grains, etc., and the amount of insulin my body makes each day is quite low.

Seventh – I now keep a food/symptom diary and follow a four-day food rotation.

Which is better – food or supplements? And which supplements should I be taking?

While there may be benefits in supplements, they are not without risks. Supplements are not regulated by the FDA. There are many reports of supplements not containing what the label claims. In addition, there are problems with purity and contamination. If the herbs or foods listed on the label are not grown on organic farms, there is a risk of heavy metal contamination (also present in non-organic food). Since the food source of the nutrient gets highly concentrated in the making of the supplement, those previously trace levels of contamination can become quite high. Another important difference is that nearly every study has shown that the whole food is associated with superior nutritional outcomes. That is likely because we absorb nutrients better when they are in food. Higher blood levels are consistently seen in comparison to food versus supplementation.

Also, in food we get the additional hundreds of other phytonutrients, all of which are likely playing contributory roles in health. I eat approximately 700 to 1000 grams of kale each day, which is filled with many different phytonutrients which have been shown to very favorably impact mitochondrial function. To consume a similar amount of critical micronutrients via supplements I would need to take 700 or more one gram tablets a day! I think that explains why I can notice a decline in energy and mental clarity if I don't eat kale for a few days, but not if I skip taking supplements.

155

As a result, I have personally focused much more on using food to get the necessary micronutrients for my mitochondria and the generation of neurotransmitters and myelin. The supplements that we suggest most often in our clinics are the following: a probiotic, multi-mineral/ multivitamin, B vitamins, fish oil, and co-enzyme Q.

What parameters should be used for electrical stimulation?
While I have been continuously experimenting on myself with electrical stimulation, I do not have data on the use of electrical stimulation in others with MS. The reference book *Application of Muscle/ Nerve Stimulation in Health and Disease* has the most comprehensive discussion of the use of electrical stimulation for health and fitness applications. The authors also discussed the limited literature that is available about the use of electrical stimulation in the setting of neurological and neuromuscular diseases. I refer all who want information on specific parameters to this reference. Those who wish to try neuromuscular electrical stimulation should work with a professional to maximize the benefit and ensure that you are not harming yourself inadvertently.

Mercury – isn't that more important than food in progressive MS?
I get this question a lot — the reality is that I do not know. I have learned that the diet I advocate supports the removal of heavy metals in the body. Mercury is toxic to the brain and spinal cord and certainly may play a role in those with progressive MS. Most likely there are many paths that lead to progressive MS, including lack of micronutrients (diet), mitochondrial dysfunction, viral infection, and toxic exposures—coupled with our unique biochemical individuality, courtesy of our DNA.

I do know that the food we eat is capable of turning on the genes that rev up inflammation or those that dampen inflammation. Food can either increase the stress on mitochondria or facilitate better-functioning mitochondria. Food can either make it easier or harder for the body to remove the toxins stored in our fat and in our brain.

While I think food had a major impact on my improvement, I remind all who read this book that your circumstances are different from mine. The things that worked so wonderfully for me have to be thoughtfully applied to your circumstances. I encourage you to talk to your doctors, nurses, and family as much as possible about your ideas of what may help you improve and maximize your health.

Do you think your food recommendations would help those with other neurological or psychological problems?

Improving the micronutrient content of the diet will help anyone who has an illness that has affected the brain. Less than ten percent of Americans eat an adequate amount of omega-3 fatty acids, and the vast majority of Americans eat less than three servings of vegetables and fruits each day. Improving the amount of fruits and vegetables and increasing the omega-3 fatty acid intake has shown to be helpful for children with attention deficit disorder, rage issues, mood issues, and behavior problems. The same has been shown to be helpful for Alzheimer's and Parkinson's patients.

Would your food recommendations help people with diabetes or other autoimmune disorders?

Improving the health of mitochondria and providing more of the amino acids, essential fatty acids, vitamins, and minerals will improve most health problems. Such a diet should be helpful for most autoimmune disorders and chronic diseases of all types. In our primary care clinics, we have many patients with diabetes, heart disease, autoimmune diseases, and mental health issues who have had significant improvement of their chronic diseases when they implemented the nine cups of vegetables and fruit each day. (See page 271 for more information on diabetic conditions.)

What kind of bicycle do you ride?

I ride a Day 6® bicycle. It has several features that are quite helpful. Since my back muscles were weak, I knew that I needed a bike that would allow me to sit upright. The Day 6 bike not only has the rider sitting upright, it also has a back rest. Since my hip flexors were also weak, I needed a bike that did not require me to lift my leg over a high cross bar. The Day 6 bike is cut low so that step through is easy. The seat is low enough to the ground that the rider can have both feet on the ground while sitting on the bike seat.

Another useful feature with the Day 6 is that an electric motor can be added on to the bike, when you purchase the bicycle, or you can have a bike mechanic add it to the bicycle any time. The motor augments your pedaling. The beauty of adding the electric motor has been that I can go biking with my family and they don't feel like they are waiting on me. It has also made it easier for me to bike to work and to the store. I still get an aerobic workout, but it's easier to commute on my bike when the ride takes 25 minutes instead of an hour. More information about the Day 6 and the electric version of the Day 6 can be found on the Web: **http://www. day6bicycles.com/**

DreamE Electric Bicycles (Day 6 with an electric motor): **http://www. day6bicycles.com/dreamE.html.**

What about those who can't chew or need tube feedings?
There are a variety of reasons why people might not be able to chew, such as having dentures or other dental problems. Other issues include tube feeding or having a small pouch for a stomach following gastric bypass surgery. In all of these circumstances, good options include smoothies and pureed soups and stews. One can use a high-speed blender to make these. I use a Vitamix. This allows me to make smoothies using fruits, nuts, brewer's yeast, and soy milk or other nut-based milks. The result is packed with nutrition and protein. Any of the soups or stews in this book can be put through a high-speed blender or Vitamix.

Diabetes and Other Auto-immune Conditions
I am often asked if the foods I recommend are good for people with diabetes. The answer is yes. The American Diabetes Association recommends a set number of grams of carbohydrates with each meal. Remember, vegetables and fruit have carbohydrates and you can fulfill your carbohydrate requirements through non-starchy vegetables/fruit and have more micronutrients, with more volume of food and less hunger.

My advice for anyone with diabetes is to increase your micronutrient intake through food. Emphasize non-starchy vegetables, lean sources of protein, and whole fruit. Be cautious using starchy vegetables, and minimize white flour and sugar. Increased omega-3 fatty acid intake (fish or flax seed) improves the body's ability to use insulin, and lowers the triglyceride levels, which are often high in those with diabetes.

The Glycemic Index refers to how quickly the blood sugar rises once you eat the food. Maintaining a low glycemic index lowers the amount of insulin your body needs.

Insulin Problems
High insulin levels lead to high levels of inflammation. Anyone with a large amount of belly fat, as evidenced by a waist that is greater than one's hips, probably has high insulin levels, high inflammation levels, and the begin-

ning of insulin resistance. With time, those individuals are high risk of becoming diabetic. What you eat can either worsen the insulin resistance or improve it.

A high-carbohydrate diet leads to a demand for high levels of insulin. A low glycemic index diet leads to a much lower demand for insulin. Therefore, a diet with a lower glycemic index lowers the amount of insulin needed to control blood sugar. Diets high in non-starchy vegetables, lean protein, and whole fruit are low glycemic index diets. They are great for someone with diabetes, great for someone with pre-diabetes, and excellent for anyone who has a lot of belly fat.

Protein has very low insulin demand. Omega-3 fatty acids improve the body's ability to use insulin. Green and other non-starchy vegetables have a low insulin demand.

In general, starchy vegetables, like potatoes, have a high insulin demand. The amount of insulin needed will depend on how the food is prepared. The more thoroughly cooked the food, the higher the glycemic index and the higher the demand for insulin. The following food groups are ranked in order to illustrate the relative amount of insulin required in response to eating those foods.

Protein=low insulin demand
Raw vegetables = modest insulin demand
Whole fruit = modest insulin demand
Boiled, mashed vegetables = moderately high insulin demand
White flour = high insulin demand
Fruit juice = higher insulin demand
Sugar = highest of all insulin demand

Resources for more glycemic index information:

http://www.diabetesnet.com/diabetes_food_diet/glycemic_index.php
http://www.southbeach-diet-plan.com/glycemicfoodchart.htm

For those who have other autoimmune conditions, a diet rich in micro-nutrients is likely to be very helpful at lowering the levels of inflammation and the amount of oxidative stress that is happening as part of the illness. As always, check with your personal physician for specific guidance on how these ideas interact with your specific medical issues.

Summary

We know that the food we eat is capable of turning genes on that rev up inflammation or that dampen inflammation. Food can either increase the stress on mitochondria or facilitate better-functioning mitochondria. Food can either make it easier or harder for the body to remove the toxins in our bodies.

While I think food had a major impact on my improvement, I remind all who read this book that your circumstances are different than mine. The things that worked so wonderfully for me have to be thoughtfully applied to your circumstances. I encourage you to talk to your doctors, nurses, and family as much as possible about your ideas of what may help you improve and maximize your health.

Food matters. If you can, grow some of your own food. Buy organic. Try eliminating the most common offenders — gluten, eggs, milk, and peanuts (legumes). If you are vegetarian and depend on soy and beans for your protein, you may elect to continue eating legumes. In that case, be mindful that you may have a soy or legume food allergy. Food testing may be necessary for you to identify which vegetarian proteins sources will work for you. Keep a food symptom diary. Try an elimination diet with a four-day food rotation. Consult with a Functional Medicine health care practitioner, nutritionist, or other healthcare provider familiar with elimination diets and food allergies. Exercise can help increase the brain growth factors and speed healing. However, without the needed micronutrients and lower levels of inflammation, you won't get far. The quality of the food and the avoidance of foods to which you are sensitive can make a big difference in your ability to improve.

Electrical therapy is a method to facilitate rehabilitation. It is not likely to restore normal walking or strength without finding a way to lower the inflammation and damage that is occurring in your brain and spinal cord. It is a way to speed gains in strength once you figure out how to cool the fires of inflammation that are occurring in your brain and spinal cord.

Chapter Eleven
CONCLUSION

The vast majority of relapsing–remitting MS patients will convert to secondary progressive MS within twenty-five years. Ten percent of MS patients start as primary progressive. Thus, it is important to all families whose lives have been touched by MS to evaluate what they can do to slow the progression of this disease and stay ambulatory as long as possible.

Present treatments have all been focused on the inflammatory component of MS even though, in progressive MS, the evidence points more to degeneration than inflammation. However, the disease is bleak once it has converted to the progressive MS phase, because there is only minimally effective medicine at that point. Physicians wanting to help patients maintain their function as long as possible are often willing to offer the potent immune-modulating drugs like Tysabri, even though there is little data supporting its use in primary or secondary progressive MS.

It is too early to know if the interventions that were so successful for me will be as effective in others. It will be a long time before we can scientifically prove that my results are reproducible in others. Although we are developing a pilot study to test these interventions in others with primary and secondary progressive MS, several hurdles must be crossed.

First, although my results are dramatic and inspiring to all who suffer from a progressive form of MS, as an experiment it was poorly designed. That is because I tried many new interventions at once. That makes it impossible to know which interventions were required, and which offered nothing but additional cost and potential side effects. A well-designed scientific experiment tests one thing at a time. That way, it is easier to know which interventions helped or failed to help. Being that precise allows us to better understand the basic mechanisms involved. Unfortunately, such an approach does not support the synergistic application of multiple interventions that would likely complement one another. It also means doing one study for several years, analyzing the data, and then designing the next step. Science is a long, slow process of building gradually upon our current knowledge.

As I watched myself decline, I knew there was no effective treatment. The clinical studies were all about relapsing-remitting MS, in part because progressive MS was so resistant to treatment. As a result, I turned to articles about the basic science of neurodegenerative diseases of the brain. I studied the literature, devised my own theories, and tested them on myself. Physicians have done that before when faced with a problem that needed an urgent answer that cannot wait for the usual incremental, plodding, but (usually) effective approach to scientific inquiry. Doing that has always required confidence in your own theories in order to be willing to take the chance and undergo the risk.

Now that I have achieved success in myself, the next step is replicating what happened to me in others. If we are successful, my basic science colleagues will use a step-by-step process to understand more precisely the mechanisms of my success. In the meantime, those of you with MS can review what I have written; discuss the interventions with your family and your physicians to decide what steps, if any, you wish to try. Those of you who have other neurological or psychological disorders may want to do the same thing, because improving the health of your brain's mitochondria is likely to improve most neurological and psychological disorders.

What about everyone else who has a chronic disease? We have an epidemic of chronic diseases that are striking our children at younger and younger ages. At the same time, we, as a society, have been providing less and less nutrition to our mitochondria. Ample evidence exists that eating more fruits and vegetables helps nearly every chronic disease, such as high blood pressure, heart disease, asthma, arthritis, and diabetes. It also lowers the risk of all forms of cancer.

Our grandmothers were right. We should probably all be eating three or more cups of fruits and vegetables with every meal, and liver once a week. Likely such an approach would have the most dramatic impact on lowering healthcare costs for the country—at a fraction of the cost of providing universal access to physicians and prescriptions.

Hippocrates, the ancient Greek physician whose oath I took in 1982, said to his students, "Let good, wholesome food be thy medicine." I don't remember ever having been told that during medical school. Or maybe I just forgot, because I was busy memorizing for the next test.

Now I see his wisdom. I wish more physicians, nurses, coaches, teachers, and young and old people could learn how mitochondria make ATP, and how food matters in that process. We need to teach everyone, from children to grandparents, that food can heal, at least in part. By eating a diet rich in micronutrients, we can achieve greater levels of health and vigor than doctors can achieve by prescribing medicines. We need to follow Hippocrates' advice and remember the critical role of food in health and disease. It is, in fact, possible to stop and even reverse much of the damage that has been done to our brains and spinal cord. Hippocrates' recommendation to his students is still the best advice, both for patients and student doctors.

Dr. Terry Wahls

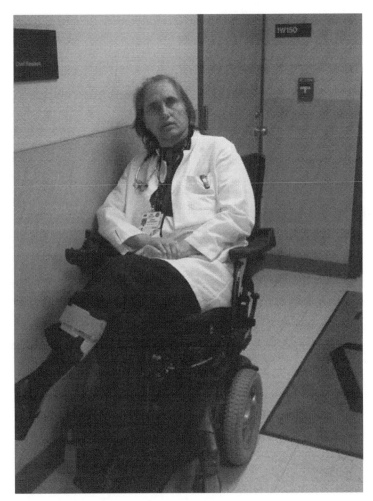

Dr. Wahls in clinic, October 2007.

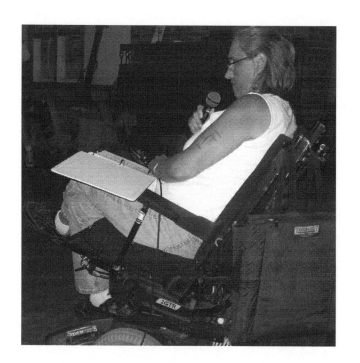
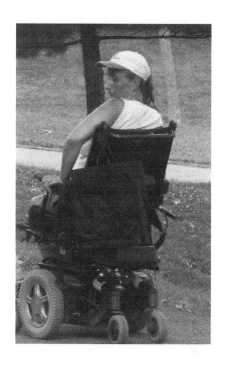

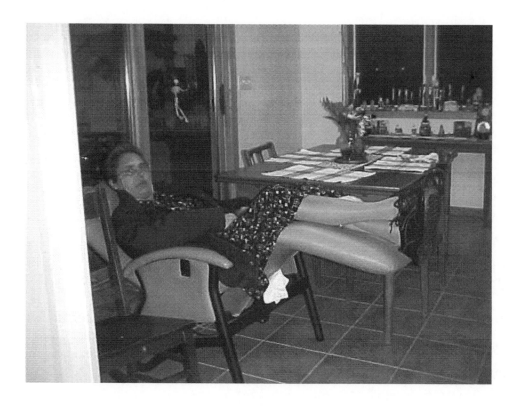

Dr. Terry Wahls
October 1, 2008

Right: Dr. Wahls with her Day 6 bicycle, October 2008.

Below: Dr. Wahls after completing a trail ride in the Canadian Rockies, October 2009.

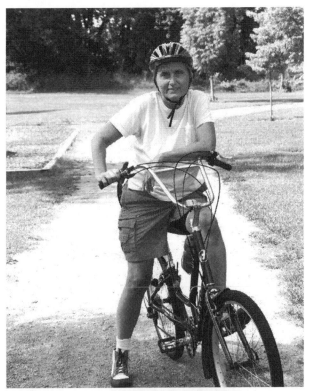

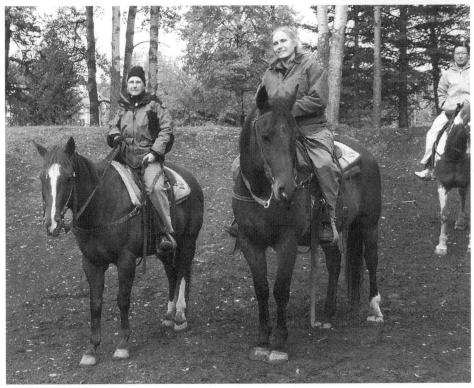

NUTRIENT AND FUNCTION CHART

Nutrient or growth factor	Dosage upper limit	Food source or intervention *(organic preferred)*	Function in the brain or mitochondria
B vitamins		Found in cooked greens, mushrooms, nutritional yeast	Helps to provide energy to the brain cell.
Thiamine B1	Up to 100 mg/day	Sunflower seeds, tuna, black beans, mushrooms, nutritional yeast, cooked or raw greens	Used to help make myelin. Can help with focus, mood, impulse control, and learning.
Riboflavin B2	Up to 200 mg/day	Almonds, organ meat, soy nuts, yogurt, mackerel, cooked greens, mushrooms	Helps provide energy (ATP) to the brain cell.
Niacinamide B3	Up to 500 mg/day	Liver, tuna, salmon, shrimp, tofu, mushrooms, potatoes with skin	Helps provide energy (ATP) to the brain cell.
Methyl Cobolamin B12 (methyl cobolamin is preferred over cyanocobolamin)	Up to 1000 mcg/day	Fish, liver, seafood, beef, egg yolks, blue-green algae, nutritional yeast	Used to help make myelin. Can help with focus, mood, impulse control, and learning. Methyl forms are more consistently absorbed and utilized by the body

Warning: Vegetarians are more at risk for low B12 levels

Nutrient or growth factor	Dosage upper limit	Food source or intervention *(organic preferred)*	Function in the brain or mitochondria
Vitamin D	Up to 2000 inter-national units (IU)/ day	Sunshine, but not so much that you burn.	Helps depression and anxiety. Several studies have shown that 4000 IU and 10000 IU daily have decreased MS activity.

Warning: Doses higher than 2000 IU should be supervised by your physician.

Nutrient or growth factor	Dosage upper limit	Food source or intervention *(organic preferred)*	Function in the brain or mitochondria
Folate *(methyl folate may be needed to overcome enzyme inefficiencies)*	Up to 800 mcg day	Green leaves, organ meat, asparagus	Important in the gener-ation of neurotrans-mitters, myelin, removal of toxins from the body. Methyl folate is more consistently absorbed and utilized by the body than regular folate.

Warning: If you take a B complex vitamin and in addition to the methyl folate you may get too much folate.

Nutrient or growth factor	Dosage upper limit	Food source or intervention *(organic preferred)*	Function in the brain or mitochondria
Multivitamin/ Multi-mineral sources		Leafy greens like spinach, beet greens, collards or kale	Helps provide energy (ATP) to the brain cell.
Coenzyme Q	200 mg (1200 mg for Parkinson's patients)	Liver, gizzards, tongue, heart, one serving per week OR 1-2 tablespoon nuts and seeds / brewer's or nutritional yeast, also green leafy vegetables	Helps provide energy (ATP) to the brain cell.
Iodine	¼ to 1 teaspoon dried seaweed/ day	Kelp, dulse, or other dried seaweed, shellfish, and sea food.	Helps provide support to making myelin and the excretion of toxins.

Warning: Iodine may affect the amount of thyroid medication needed. Can also unmask an overactive thyroid. Monitor thyroid hormone blood levels.

Nutrient or growth factor	Dosage upper limit	Food source or intervention *(organic preferred)*	Function in the brain or mitochondria
Magnesium	500 mg elemental	Pumpkin seeds, sesame seeds, cabbage family vegetables	Helps mood, impulsivity, and chronic pain.
Theanine	500 mg	Green tea	Helps focus and calming
Taurine	1 to grams	Fish and Shell fish	Key ingredient for neurotransmitters. Helps with pain, anxiety, and other mood disorders.
Sulfur-containing vegetables	3 cups /day 300 to 1000 grams	Cabbage (kale, collards, radishes, broccoli, cauliflower etc.) onion (garlic, leeks, onions, shallots)	Helps with the generation of neurotransmitters.
Antioxidants	3 cups / day 300 grams	Intensely colored vegetables/ fruits, such as beets, carrots, squash, berries, peaches	Helps mitochondria get rid of toxic trash (free radicals) that is made while converting food into ATP, used for energy.

Nutrient or growth factor	Dosage upper limit	Food source or intervention (*organic preferred*)	Function in the brain or mitochondria
Resveratrol	Up 200 mg / day	Purple grape juice, blue-black berries, and fruits. It is thought to be the protective part of red wine	Potent anti-oxidant; useful as an anti-aging compound, as found in several animal models of aging.
N acetylcysteine	1 to 2 grams	Leafy greens, spinach, beet greens, cabbage, kale, collards, broccoli, cauliflower, radishes, onions, leeks, garlic, shallots	Key ingredient for neurotransmitters. Helps with impulse control, irritability, and other mood problems. Also helps with chronic pain.
Omega-3 fatty acids			
Fish oil	1 to 4 grams / day	Salmon or mackerel 2+ times a week (canned wild is good) *OR* DHA-enriched eggs	Used to make myelin. Can help with focus, mood, impulse control, and learning.
Flax Oil or Hemp Oil	1 to 2 tablespoons/ day	You can't cook with flax oil – but you can mix it with rice vinegar and soy sauce and use as a salad dressing on greens	Used to make myelin. Can help with focus, mood, impulse control, and learning.

Warning: Omega-3 may cause bleeding / bruising if taken with aspirin or other medicines to thin the blood

Nutrient or growth factor	Dosage upper limit	Food source or intervention (*organic preferred*)	Function in the brain or mitochondria
Trace minerals	¼ to 1 teaspoon kelp or algae daily has been helpful	Sea weed, algae	Minerals are important parts of many enzymes. They are also important in the de-toxification of heavy metals and synthetic compounds.
Creatine Monohydrate	1 teaspoon	Fish, shellfish, venison, and other wild game meats	Helps with the generation of ATP (energy) and may decrease muscle wasting.
Alpha Lipoic Acid	600mg	Spinach, broccoli, beef, yeast (particularly brewer's yeast), and certain organ meats (such as the kidney and heart)	May help reduce pain, burning, itching, tingling, and numbness in people who have nerve damage (per-ipheral neuropathy) caused by diabetes. Has been used with L-carnitine and found (in animal studies) to be helpful in improving mito-chondria health to prolong life.

Warning: Trace minerals – Watch thyroid hormone levels when using sea-weed, amount of thyroid medication needed may change. May cause the thyroid to become overactive.
Creatine Monohydrate requires plenty of hydration to avoid kidney stones.

Nutrient or growth factor	Dosage upper limit	Food source or intervention *(organic preferred)*	Function in the brain or mitochondria
L carnitine	500 mg	Red meat, wild game	Used with Lipoic acid in anti-aging studies to improve mitochondrial health and prolong life.
Probiotics (beneficial bacteria for the colon)		Fermented foods	Helpful in displacing potential harmful bacteria that produce toxins, which can be harmful to the body. Also helpful in digesting food into specific micronutrients and vitamins.

Warning: Probiotics — Read the labels. You may wish to avoid those that use cereal grasses in the formulation.

Nutrient or growth factor	Dosage upper limit	Food source or intervention *(organic preferred)*	Function in the brain or mitochondria
Nerve growth factors			
Physical activity		Walking, climbing stairs at work, parking further from destination	Stimulate the brain to repair damage. Also very good for mood.
Learning new physical activities		Activities involving hand-eye coordination, such as juggling, knitting, or a new sport	Stimulate the brain to repair damage. Also very good for mood.
Mental learning		Reading, solving puzzles, learning something new	Stimulates the brain to repair damage. Also very good for mood.

Please remember to always discuss with your personal physician **PRIOR** to starting any vitamins or supplements, as your personal health circumstances may make these vitamins or supplements harmful to you.

ABBREVIATIONS

Abbreviation	Term
ATP	Adenosine triphosphate
DHA	Docosohexanoic acid
EPA	Eicosopentanoic acid
FADH	Flavin adenosine dinucleotide
FES	Functional electrical stimulation
GABA	Gamma amino Butyric Acid
HDL	High density lipoprotein, or good cholesterol
NAC	N-acetyl cysteine
NADH	Niacinamide adenosine dinucleotide
NMES	Neuromuscular electrical stimulation
TENS	Transcutaneous electrical stimulation
SNPs	Single Nucleotide Polymorphism

Sample Menus

DAY 1	Morning smoothie (*soy milk, green tea, banana, cardamom, chlorella*)	red cabbage wedge, carrots, apple	kale, garlic salad (*with hemp oil + lime juice dressing*), cup bone broth, beef roast in bone
DAY 2	Hot Morning smoothie (*almond milk, cocoa, cinnamon, flax meal, peach*)	spinach salad, green beans, black grapes	soup (*curried peanut butter greens*), bok choy salad (*with flax oil, rice vinegar salad dressing*), bone broth
DAY 3	Morning Smoothie (*rasp-berries, hemp milk*)	collard, onion, greens salad, turnip slices, orange	collards with black-eyed peas, carrots, celery, bone broth, black cherries
DAY 4	Morning smoothie (*hot yerba mate, spirulina, cloves, banana, rice milk*)	romaine salad, apples, blueberries	romaine, avocado, and walnut salad (*with hemp oil, lime juice, cilantro dressing*) lamb chop, cup bone broth
DAY 5	Morning smoothie (*green grapes, kale leaf, apple juice, sunflower seeds, cinnamon*)	kale salad, carrots, celery	soup (*kale, potato, yam, coconut milk with sausage*), beet salad
DAY 6	Morning smoothie (*aronia or cran-berries, nutmeg, soy milk*)	sushi, seaweed salad, pear on side	fish soup (*clams, mussels, shrimp, onion, leeks, tomatoes*), spinach salad
DAY 7	Morning smoothie (*red cabbage, cranberry juice, ice, flax oil*)	humus, turnip slices, squash slices	roast chicken with squash filberts, beet salad, steamed mustard greens, bone broth

DAY 8	Morning smoothie (*blueberries, spinach, sunflower seeds*)	red pepper, squash, radishes, pomegranate juice	grilled chicken, leaf lettuce salad, fresh onions, muskmelon
DAY 9	Morning smoothie (*romaine, pear, apple juice*) apple	beet salad, carrots, pear, pumpkin seeds	sandwich on gluten-free bread (*canned salmon, onion, celery salad, with romaine*) avocado salad, carrot
DAY 10	Morning Smoothie (*aronia, red cabbage, banana, soy milk*)	asparagus, red pepper, summer squash salad, hummus	black eyed peas, mustard greens or collards, onion soup
DAY 11	Morning smoothie (*cranberries, apple juice, hemp milk*) pear	kale, garlic, onion salad, apple, blueberries	liver, mushroom and onions, kale, garlic salad, peaches
DAY 12	Morning smoothie (*black cherries, almond milk*)	strawberries, spinach salad, sunflower seeds	grilled hamburger (*1 cup minced fresh garden herbs mixed into 1 lb of meat prior to grilling*) grilled yams, sweet peppers, mush-rooms, greens, spinach, strawberry salad
DAY 13	Morning smoothie (*green grapes, kale, lemon juice, sunflower seeds*)	clam chowder, coconut milk base, mushroom, onions, leeks, yam	fish taco (*with corn tortillas, minced red cabbage*) black berries
DAY 14	Morning smoothie (*spirulina, green tea, flax meal, black grapes*)	spaghetti squash, filberts, collard green salad, cashews	eggplant, garlic, peanut butter dip, raw carrots, veggie slices, grilled pork chop, steamed collards

Gluten free resources: There are numerous recipes and products that allow you to make breads, pancakes, cereals, pies, and pasta—all gluten free. We recommend limited intake of gluten free grains, but it does make the transition to gluten free much easier. Visit *www.celiac.com* and *http://www.breadsfromanna.com/recipes*. (Anna Sobaski, creator of Breads From Anna®, is an Iowa City chef who has gluten free mixes. Our family has used them quite successfully!)

DAILY LOG

ACTIVITIES AND FOOD

	Minutes		Minutes
Skin contact: Goal 10 min		Quiet time: Goal 20 minutes	
Massage		Prayer	
Stroking		Meditation	
Learning: Goal 15 minutes		Guided Imagery	
Nintendo DS Brain Age		Yoga	
Sudoku		Tai Chi	
Crossword Puzzles		Nature	
	Amounts		**Amounts**
Cups cruciferous, onion, mushroom		Servings plant protein	
Cups bright colors		Servings animal protein	
Cups other vegetables		Servings minerals	
Cups approved milks		Servings essential fats	
Servings of foods not approved		Servings non-gluten grains	

Cruciferous/Greens Goal 3 cups	cups	Onion/Mushroom Goal 1 cup	cups	Blue/Black Goal 1 cup	cups
Kale		Onion /shallots		Blue potato	
Collards		Leeks		Black grapes	
Mustard greens		Chives		Blue berries	
Turnip greens		Mushrooms		Pomegranate	
Green Cabbage		Garlic (# of cloves)		Red beets	
Red cabbage		**Other vegetables**		Mulberries	
Chinese cabbage		Eggplant / peppers		Elderberries	
Broccoli		Artichoke / avocado		Black berries	
Cauliflower		Fennel /celiac		Plum	
Brussels sprouts		Parsnips		**Yellow/Orange** Goal 1 cup	
Radishes		Asparagus			
Turnips		Green beans /peas		Carrot	
Kohlrabi		corn		Squash	
Broccoli		Summer squash /okra		Peaches	
Bok Choy		**Total other vegetables**		Oranges	
Leaf lettuce		**Red** Goal 1 cup		Pumpkin	
Beet greens		Tomatoes		Yellow beets	
Spinach		Red pepper		Muskmelon	
Romaine		Watermelon		Pineapple	
Other greens		Strawberries		Yams / sweet potatoes	
Turnips/ rutabaga		Red beets		Orange peppers	
Other		Red berries			
Total cruciferous/ onion/ mushroom		**Total brightly colored**			

Minerals ¼ to 1 teaspoons		Animal Protein goal 4 oz.		Other fruits vegetables	
Dried sea weed *teaspoons*		Fish, shell fish *Wild/Farm*	W F	Dried Greens *teaspoons*	
Dried Kelp *teaspoons*		Lamb *grass fed*	Y N	Algae	
Sea salt *teaspoons*		Poultry *free range*	Y N	**Non gluten grains** *circle* – rice, millet, oatmeal, buckwheat bread, cereal, pasta –	
Nutritional yeast *teaspoons*		Beef *grass fed*	Y N		
Bone broth *(cups)*		Pork *pasture*	Y N		
Total minerals		Total animal protein			
Plant Protein		**Approved Milks**		**Foods Not On food list**	
Walnut, almond, pecan, brazil nut, filbert, nut butter, pumpkin seeds - *tablespoons*		Soy milk		Grains with Gluten *circle* Rye, wheat, barley, bread, cereal, pasta	
Gluten free soy sauce -*tablespoons* or 4 oz. tofu		Almond milk		Pastries, cakes, pies, deserts	
Legumes / beans		Filbert milk		Dairy , cheese, milk, ice cream	
Total plant protein		Rice milk		French fries	
Total essential fats		Total approved milks		Candy	
Essential fats/oils		**Spices** *circle* - cinnamon, cloves, cardamom, nutmeg, turmeric, ginger, parsley, sage, rosemary, thyme, basil, oregano, cumin, coriander, bay, black pepper, fennel, fenugreek		Other	
Flax/ Hemp Oil *tablespoons*				Total foods not recommended	
Fish oil capsules				Total non gluten grains	
Krill oil capsules					

180

Note: 1 cup = small banana, apple, chopped raw vegetables, ½ cup cooked vegetables, 2 cups leafy greens (i.e. spinach, romaine or kale), 1 teaspoon spirulina or chlorella or blue green algae.

Circle foods eaten not on diet: eggs, dairy, gluten grains(wheat, barley, rye), other grains, fast food, French fries, candy, liquid oils other than hemp or flax oil

Rate the following by circling the appropriate response
Pain- *none/ minimal, mild, moderate, severe, total*
Fatigue- *none/ minimal, mild, moderate,   severe, total*
Hours slept in previous 24 hrs_____

Figure 1: Detoxification Pathways

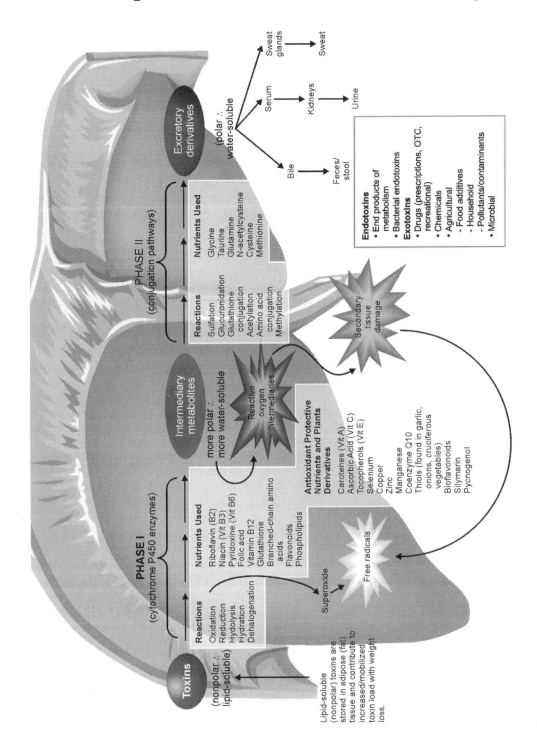

Liver detoxification pathways and supportive nutrients

Figure 2: Nutrients Supporting Detoxification

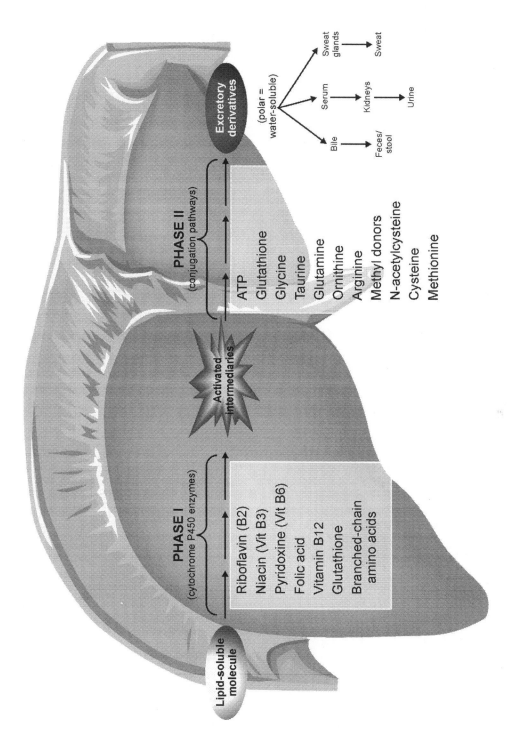

Supportive Nutrients for Detoxification Pathways

Figure 3: Foods Supporting Detoxification

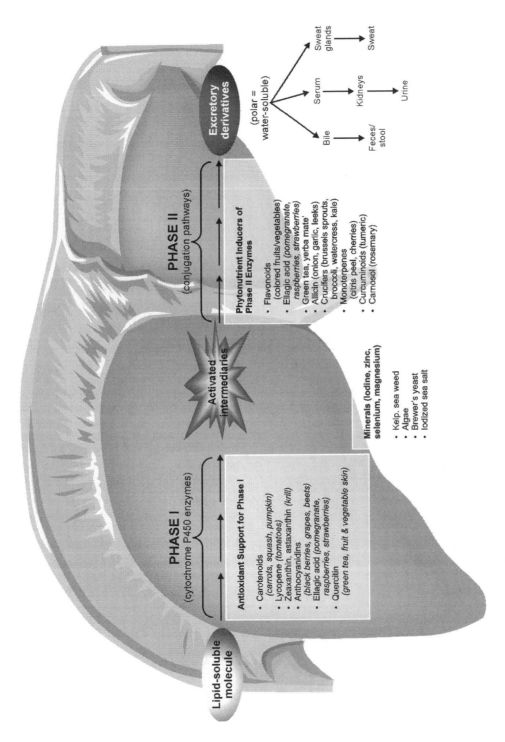

Supportive Foods for Detoxification Pathways

Figure 4: The Role of Food Allergies in Chronic Disease

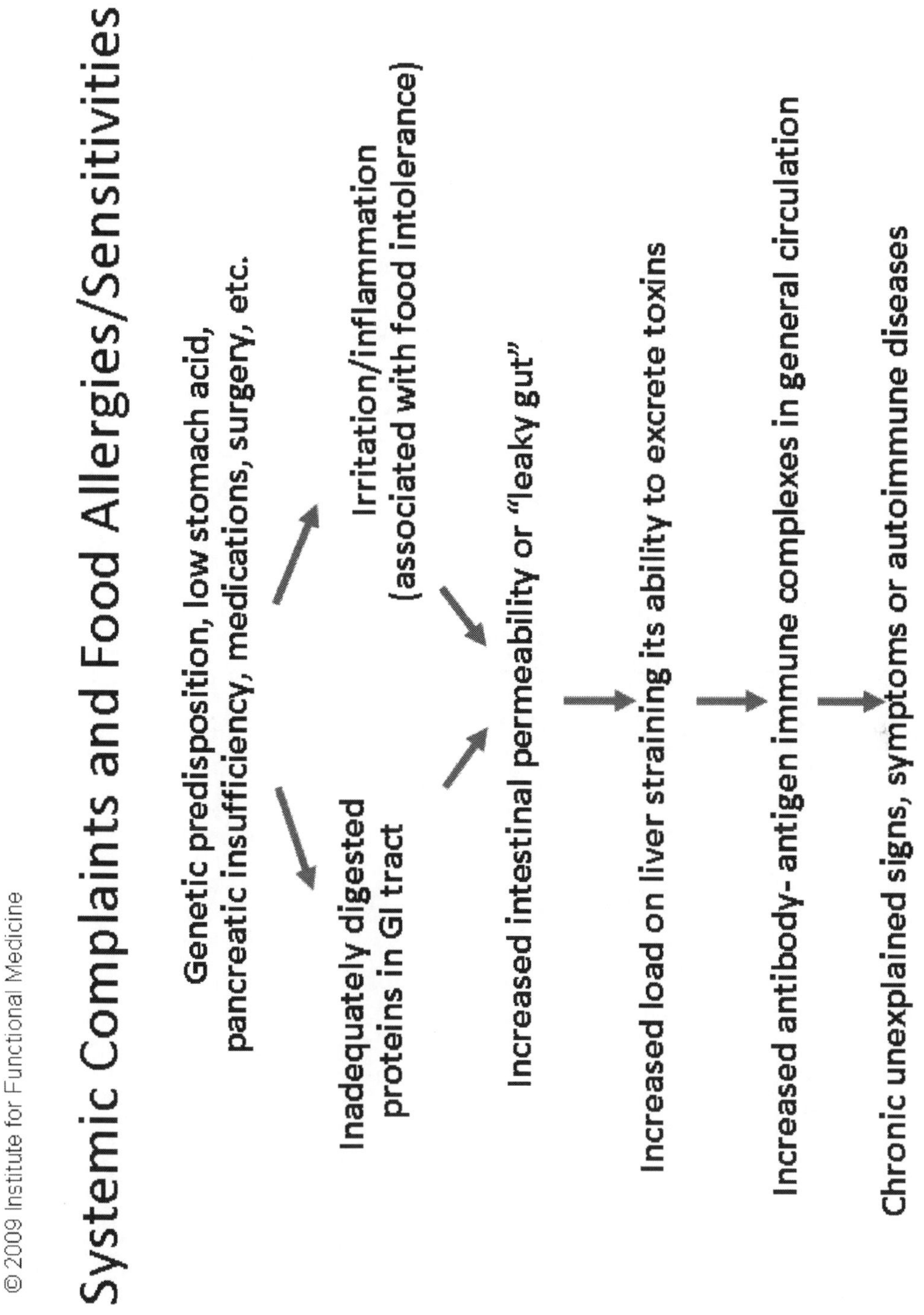
© 2009 Institute for Functional Medicine
Systemic Complaints and Food Allergies/Sensitivities
Genetic predisposition, low stomach acid, pancreatic insufficiency, medications, surgery, etc.
Irritation/inflammation (associated with food intolerance)
Inadequately digested proteins in GI tract
Increased intestinal permeability or "leaky gut"
Increased load on liver straining its ability to excrete toxins
Increased antibody- antigen immune complexes in general circulation
Chronic unexplained signs, symptoms or autoimmune diseases

Figure 5: Conventional Medicine and Functional Medicine Approaches to Diagnosis and Treatment of Disease

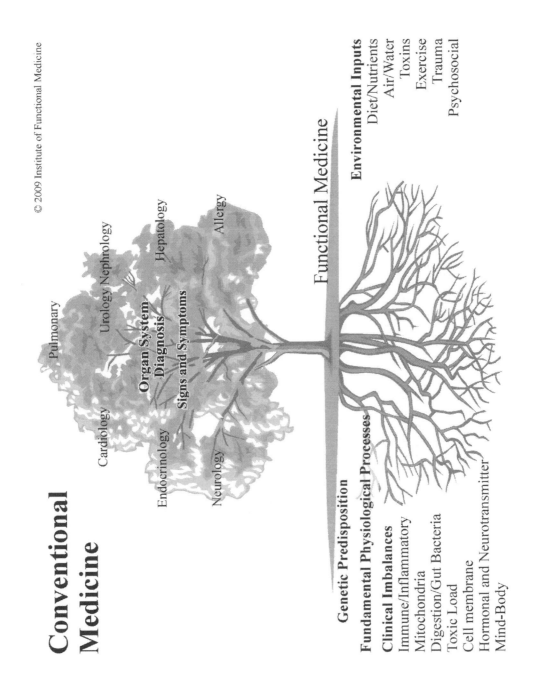

© 2009 Institute of Functional Medicine

Conventional medicine uses medication to control symptoms. Functional medicine focuses on improving environmental inputs to rebalance the workings of the mitochondria and cell (clinical imbalances). Functional medicine does not consider genetic predisposition to be insurmountable, i.e., with improved environmental inputs health can often be restored

Glossary

Adenosine tri-phosphate
The molecule cells use to store energy, which can be used to have controlled chemical reactions, to make proteins, antibodies, and other structures important to life; often referred to as ATP.

Aerobic
An environment with oxygen, usually referring to generating ATP in the presence of oxygen and mitochondria.

Algae
Single-celled marine plants that are high in omega 3 fatty acids, protein, and chlorophyll.

Anaerobic
An environment without oxygen, usually referring to having to generate ATP without oxygen and without mitochondria.

Antioxidants
A chemical that the cell can use to capture a free radical before it does any damage to other parts of the cell.

Aspartame
The chemical name for NutraSweet®; used as a sweetener. It can increase the levels of specific neurotransmitter molecules in the brain, which can, at times, become toxic.

Axons
Part of the connecting portion or "wiring" between the neurons or brain cells.

Baclofen
A drug that is often given to combat muscle spasms. One of the effects it has on the brain is to increase the levels of GABA in the brain, which help lower the excessive stimulation of brain cells.

Beta endorphins
A molecule that is generated in the brain by exercise. It is also associated

with a sense of well-being, euphoria, and lower levels of inflammation molecules.

Bio-energetics
The process by which the cell generates energy or ATP molecules that it can use to drive other work the cell must do to live.

Brain-derived neurotrophic growth factor A molecule that stimulates growth of brain cells. Exercise has been shown to increase the production of this molecule. Also called BDNF.

Celiac disease
A condition in which the individual has become allergic to gluten, a protein found it wheat. The result is damage to the small bowel, which interferes with absorption of key nutrients; often associated with psychiatric and neurological symptoms.

Chlorella
A kind of fresh-water algae that has been demonstrated to bind heavy metals in the gut and improve the body's ability to detoxify. Cell walls must be "cracked" so the body can utilize the nutrients within chlorella. Is very high in chlorophyll.

Co-enzyme Q10
A more common name for ubiquinone, which is a molecule used by the electron transport chain within the mitochondria to generate ATP.

Creatine Monohydrate
An amino acid that is used in the generation of ATP.

Cruciferous
The cabbage family of vegetables that includes collards, cabbage, kale, cauliflower, broccoli, radish, and kohlrabi.

Cytokines
A molecule that is associated with inflammation.

Dendrites
Part of the connective "wiring" between brain cells.

Depolarization
Part of the process the nerve uses to transmit information down the length of the nerve onto the next nerve.

Docosohexanoic acid
An omega-3 fatty acid that is incorporated in the lining of nerve cells; an important component of myelin or nerve cell insulation (DHA).

Eicosopentanoic acid
An omega-3 fatty acid that is incorporated in the lining of nerve cells; an important component of myelin or nerve cell insulation (EPA).

Electron transport chain
A part of the mitochondria that utilizes FADH, NADH, and ubiquinone to generate ATP for the cell.

Excito-toxicity
When certain neurotransmitters stimulate the nerve cell to excessive levels, the nerve cell is stressed at times to the point of nerve-cell death.

Experimental autoimmune encephalitis
An animal model of multiple sclerosis, which is used by scientists to understand the causes and potential treatments for MS.

Experimental optic neuritis
An animal model of optic neuritis, which is often a precursor to multiple sclerosis.

Flavin adenosine dinucleotide
A molecule used by the mitochondria to generate ATP. It is derived from riboflavin, a B vitamin.

Free radicals
A molecule that is a by-product of the generation of ATP. If it is not captured immediately by an antioxidant, the free radical will damage the mitochondria and the DNA of the cell. Free radicals are responsible for the progression of most chronic diseases and are likely key culprits in the transformation of a healthy cell into a cancerous cell.

Functional electrical stimulation
A type of electrical stimulation that is timed with a repetitive activity, such as walking or bicycling (FES).

Gabapentin
A drug that is often used in the setting of MS to control pain. It is also an effective seizure medication and is believed to work by increasing brain GABA levels.

Gamma amino butyric acid
A neurotransmitter that is the counterbalance to glutamate. It is a neuro-inhibitor and helps calm the brain, decrease pain, seizures, and spasms (GABA).

Glial growth factor
A molecule that is made in the brain and helps stimulate the growth of cells that make the myelin or lining of the nerve cell.

Glutamate
A neurotransmitter that is important in learning. It is often found in excess in conditions of chronic pain, increased muscle spasms, and neurodegenerative conditions, like multiple sclerosis. When excessive, glutamate can become toxic to brain and nerve cells.

Glutathione
An amino acid that contains sulfur and is important in the generation of neurotransmitters in the brain, especially GABA.

Incontinence
The absence of good control for bowel or bladder function, which results in accidental wetting or soiling of the individual.

Insulin-like growth factor
A molecule made in the brain in response to exercise that stimulates growth of brain cells.

Kelp
A seaweed that is an excellent source of iodine and other trace minerals.

Krebs cycle
A series of chemical reactions in the mitochondria, which convert the energy stored in glucose into energy stored in the ATP molecule.

L-carnitine
A molecule used by the mitochondria in the generation of energy.

Lipoic acid
A molecule used by the mitochondria in the generation of energy.

Melatonin
A hormone secreted by the brain in response to darkness, which supports the initiation and maintenance of sleep.

Micronutrients
Vitamins, minerals, and other molecules needed by the cells as building blocks or catalysts for healthy living.

Mitochondria
The organelle that was likely derived from ancient bacteria and since incorporated as the mitochondria within the cell. It is also the place where ATP is generated by the cell.

Monosodium glutamate
Also called MSG. A molecule that often increases the brain glutamate or aspartate levels. In some individuals, the increased glutamate causes headaches, weakness, and other neurological and psychological symptoms.

Myelin
The insulation that wraps around the axons and dendrites, which connect the neurons or brain cells to one another.

N Acetylcysteine
An amino acid that contains sulfur, important in the generation of GABA, and also a powerful antioxidant for mitochondrial health.

Nerve growth factor
A molecule in the brain that increases with exercise and stimulates the growth of brain cells and nerves.

Neuromuscular electrical stimulation
The electrical stimulation placed over the motor nerve to induce a muscular contraction. Typically, the patient adds a volitional muscle contraction on top of the electrical contraction (NMES).

Neurotransmitter
A molecule used by the nerve cells to communicate with one another. Examples include serotonin, GABA, glutamate, and others.

Niacinamide
A B vitamin important in mitochondrial function.

Niacinamide adenosine dinucleotide
A molecule that facilitates the transfer of electrons to generate ATP molecules in the mitochondria (NADH).

Norepinephrine
A neurotransmitter often increased in the setting of increased anxiety, hyper-vigilance, and attention deficit disorder.

Omega-3 fatty acid
An essential—meaning that the body cannot make it on its own—fatty acid that is part of myelin. Omega-3 fatty acids also influence the amount of inflammation in the body. Higher levels of omega-3 fatty acids decrease inflammation. Good sources include salmon, mackerel, and fish oil. Flax oil and hemp oil also contain omega-3 fatty acids.

Omega-6 fatty acids
An essential fatty acid, meaning the body cannot make it on its own. High levels of omega-6 fatty acids relative to lower levels of omega-3 fatty acids increase inflammation. Corn-fed meat has high levels of omega-6 fatty acids, and markedly diminished levels of omega-3 fatty acids.

Organic Sulfur
Amino acids that contain sulfur are important for the brain to generate neurotransmitters, especially GABA. Also important in the mitochondria as antioxidants.

Oxidative stress
When the mitochondria do not have sufficient B vitamins and antioxidants

to function properly, less ATP is generated, along with more free radicals. This shift of more free radicals per ATP molecule is called oxidative stress.

Oxidize
The chemical reaction that occurs when free radicals damage the cell structures.

Parkinson's disease
A neurodegenerative disease affecting the brain's ability to make dopamine. It leads to progressive muscle stiffness, tremors, and dementia.

Polyphenols
A plant-based molecule that acts as an antioxidant.

Primary progressive MS
Ten percent of people initially diagnosed with MS experience a relentless downhill course without acute symptoms. There are no effective treatments that prevent or reverse disability due to primary progressive MS (also called PPMS).

Relapsing-remitting MS
Also called RRMS. Eighty percent of people initially diagnosed with MS have acute relapses of MS-related symptoms, such as visual change, weakness, or pain. The nerve cells add sodium channels so that they can again transmit information, although it is somewhat slower. With time, the vast majority of RRMS patients transition into secondary MS and experience gradual worsening of symptoms without acute relapses.

Resveratrol
A potent antioxidant found in dark purple or black fruit. Has been associated with longevity.

Riboflavin
A B vitamin important in the generation of ATP within mitochondria.

Secondary progressive MS
The vast majority of patients who start with a diagnosis of RRMS will evolve into secondary progressive MS (SPMS). They will then experience a gradual worsening of MS symptoms without significant changes on brain

or spinal cord MRI.

Serotonin
A neurotransmitter involved in depression and mania.

Single Nucleotide Polymorphism
A change in the DNA in which one DNA nucleotide has been replaced with an incorrect nucleotide. The result is that the enzyme for which that portion of the DNA is the blueprint is made incorrectly.

Sodium channels
Nerves add these to their membranes to restore transmission of information down the nerve.

Spirulina
A type of fresh-water algae that binds heavy metals in the gut and improves the body's ability to detoxify. Is very high in chlorophyll.

Taurine
An amino acid that has organic sulfur, important to the generation of GABA.

Theanine
An amino acid that diminishes norepinephrine and improves focus and concentration.

Transcutaneous electrical stimulation
The use of electrical impulses over the sensory nerves to deplete some of the neurotransmitters involved in pain. Has also been used recently to improve bladder control (TENS).

Ubiquinone
Structurally similar to B vitamins. It is an important molecule in the generation of ATP through the electron transport chain.

Xenobiotic
Synthetic or man-made compound that interacts with living cells. Must be excreted through urine, sweat, or bile to be removed from the body.

Internet sources for less-expensive, ultra-refined omega-3 fatty acids, vitamins, nutritional supplements, and teas are: **www.SwansonVitamins.com, www.iHerb.com, www.bio-aleternative.net, puprebulk.com,** and **www.vitacost.com**. Readers are reminded to be cautious with the purchase of nutritional supplements and products, as they are not regulated by the federal Food and Drug Administration. As a result, the quality and purity of the substances is not regulated and therefore may be unreliable. Look for companies whose products are compliant with Good Manufactguring Processes as verified by a third party audit. Always discuss with your personal health care provider prior to starting vitamins or supplements, or making a major change in your diet, as your personal situation may require a very different approach than has been discussed in this book.

Reference List

(1) Beauloye V, Zech F, Tran HT et al. Determinants of early atherosclerosis in obese children and adolescents. J Clin Endocrinol Metab 2007; 92(8):3025-3032.

(2) de Silva KS, Wickramasinghe VP, Gooneratne IN. Metabolic consequences of childhood obesity—a preliminary report. Ceylon Med J 2006; 51(3):105-109.

(3) Laron Z. Increasing incidence of childhood obesity. Pediatr Endocrinol Rev 2004; 1 Suppl 3:443-447.

(4) Pinhas-Hamiel O, Singer S, Pilpel N et al. Health-related quality of life among children and adolescents: associations with obesity. Int J Obes (Lond) 2006; 30(2):267-272.

(5) Goran MI. Metabolic precursors and effects of obesity in children: a decade of progress, 1990-1999. Am J Clin Nutr 2001; 73(2):158-171.

(6) Kovacs M, Feinberg TL, Crouse-Novak M et al. Depressive disorders in childhood. II. A longitudinal study of the risk for a subsequent major depression. Arch Gen Psychiatry 1984; 41(7):643-649.

(7) Wells VE, Deykin EY, Klerman GL. Risk factors for depression in adolescence. Psychiatr Dev 1985; 3(1):83-108.

(8) Abuissa H, Bel DS, O'Keefe JH, Jr. Strategies to prevent type 2 diabetes. Curr Med Res Opin 2005; 21(7):1107-1114.

(9) Botero D, Wolfsdorf JI. Diabetes mellitus in children and adolescents. Arch Med Res 2005; 36(3):281-290.

(10) Bray GA, Gray DS. Obesity. Part I—Pathogenesis. West J Med 1988; 149(4):429-441.

(11) James PT, Leach R, Kalamara E et al. The worldwide obesity epidemic. Obes Res 2001; 9 Suppl 4:228S-233S.

(12) Biederman J, Faraone SV. The Massachusetts General Hospital studies of gender influences on attention-deficit/hyperactivity disorder in youth and relatives. Psychiatr Clin North Am 2004; 27(2):225-232.

(13) Ireys HT, Salkever DS, Kolodner KB et al. Schooling, employment, and idleness in young adults with serious physical health conditions: effects of age, disability status, and parental education. J Adolesc Health 1996; 19(1):25-33.

(14) Kube DA, Petersen MC, Palmer FB. Attention deficit hyperactivity disorder: comorbidity and medication use. Clin Pediatr (Phila) 2002; 41(7):461-469.

(15) Sebestik J, Garralda ME. Survey of difficult to contain and treat

children and adolescents. Arch Dis Child 1996; 75(1):78–81.

(16) Al-Tahan J, Gonzalez-Gross M, Pietrzik K. B-vitamin status and intake in European adolescents. A review of the literature. Nutr Hosp 2006; 21(4):452–465

(17) Clark AJ, Mossholder S, Gates R. Folacin status in adolescent females. Am J Clin Nutr 1987; 46(2):302–306.

(18) de Carvalho MJ, Guilland JC, Moreau D et al. Vitamin status of healthy subjects in Burgundy (France). Ann Nutr Metab 1996; 40(1):24–51.

(19) Simopoulos AP. Human requirement for N-3 polyunsaturated fatty acids. Poult Sci 2000; 79(7):961–970.

(20) Simopoulos AP. Omega-3 fatty acids in health and disease and in growth and development. Am J Clin Nutr 1991; 54(3):438–463.

(21) Plaitakis A, Shashidharan P. Glutamate transport and metabolism in dopaminergic neurons of substantia nigra: implications for the pathogenesis of Parkinson's disease. J Neurol 2000; 247 Suppl 2:II25-II35.

(22) Savolainen KM, Loikkanen J, Eerikainen S et al. Glutamate-stimulated ROS production in neuronal cultures: interactions with lead and the cholinergic system. Neurotoxicology 1998; 19(4–5):669–674.

(23) Klepstad P, Maurset A, Moberg ER et al. Evidence of a role for NMDA receptors in pain perception. Eur J Pharmacol 1990; 187(3):513–518.

(24) Zorumski CF, Olney JW. Excitotoxic neuronal damage and neuropsychiatric disorders. Pharmacol Ther 1993; 59(2):145–162.

(25) Pelaez B, Blazquez JL, Pastor FE et al. Lectinhistochemistry and ultrastructure of microglial response to monosodium glutamate-mediated neurotoxicity in the arcuate nucleus. Histol Histopathol 1999; 14(1):165–174.

(26) Maher TJ, Wurtman RJ. Possible neurologic effects of aspartame, a widely used food additive. Environ Health Perspect 1987; 75:53–57.

(27) Whitehouse CR, Boullata J, McCauley LA. The potential toxicity of artificial sweeteners. AAOHN J 2008; 56(6):251–259.

(28) Drevets WC. Orbitofrontal cortex function and structure in depression. Ann N Y Acad Sci 2007; 1121:499–527.

(29) Kalia M. Neurobiological basis of depression: an update. Metabolism 2005; 54(5 Suppl 1):24–27.

(30) Kendell SF, Krystal JH, Sanacora G. GABA and glutamate systems as therapeutic targets in depression and mood disorders. Expert Opin Ther Targets 2005; 9(1):153–168.

(31) Blumberg HP, Charney DS, Krystal JH. Frontotemporal neural systems in bipolar disorder. Semin Clin Neuropsychiatry 2002; 7(4):243–254.

(32) Krystal JH, Sanacora G, Blumberg H et al. Glutamate and GABA systems as targets for novel antidepressant and mood-stabilizing treatments. Mol Psychiatry 2002; 7 Suppl 1:S71–S80.

(33) Henry PG, Russeth KP, Tkac I et al. Brain energy metabolism and neurotransmission at near-freezing temperatures: in vivo (1)H MRS study of a hibernating mammal. J Neurochem 2007; 101(6):1505–1515

(34) Perry TL, Yong VW, Bergeron C et al. Amino acids, glutathione, and glutathione transferase activity in the brains of patients with Alzheimer's disease. Ann Neurol 1987; 21(4):331-336.

(35) Albrecht J. Roles of neuroactive amino acids in ammonia neurotoxicity. J Neurosci Res 1998; 51(2):133–138.

(36) Demakova EV, Korobov VP, Lemkina LM. [Determination of gamma-aminobutyric acid concentration and activity of glutamate decarboxylase in blood serum of patients with multiple sclerosis]. Klin Lab Diagn 2003;(4):15–17.

(37) Addolorato G, Leggio L, D'Angelo C et al. Affective and psychiatric disorders in celiac disease. Dig Dis 2008; 26(2):140–148.

(38) Pynnonen PA, Isometsa ET, Aronen ET et al. Mental disorders in adolescents with celiac disease. Psychosomatics 2004; 45(4):325–335.

(39) Vaile JH, Meddings JB, Yacyshyn BR et al. Bowel permeability and CD45RO expression on circulating CD20+ B cells in patients with ankylosing spondylitis and their relatives. J Rheumatol 1999; 26(1):128–135.

(40) Yacyshyn B, Meddings J, Sadowski D et al. Multiple sclerosis patients have peripheral blood CD45RO+ B cells and increased intestinal permeability. Dig Dis Sci 1996; 41(12):2493–2498.

(41) Yacyshyn BR, Meddings JB. CD45RO expression on circulating CD19+ B cells in Crohn's disease correlates with intestinal permeability. Gastroenterology 1995; 108(1):132–137.

(42) Jew S, AbuMweis SS, Jones PJ. Evolution of the human diet: linking our ancestral diet to modern functional foods as a means of chronic disease prevention. J Med Food 2009; 12(5):925–934.

(43) Stiner MC, Barkai R, Gopher A. Cooperative hunting and meat sharing 400-200 kya at Qesem Cave, Israel. Proc Natl Acad Sci U S A 2009; 106(32):13207–13212.

(44) Jonsson T, Granfeldt Y, Ahren B et al. Beneficial effects of a Paleolithic diet on cardiovascular risk factors in type 2 diabetes: a

randomized cross-over pilot study. Cardiovasc Diabetol 2009; 8:35.

(45) Jonsson T, Ahren B, Pacini G et al. A Paleolithic diet confers higher insulin sensitivity, lower C-reactive protein and lower blood pressure than a cereal-based diet in domestic pigs. Nutr Metab (Lond) 2006; 3:39.

(46) Halperin ML, Cheema-Dhadli S, Lin SH et al. Control of potassium excretion: a Paleolithic perspective. Curr Opin Nephrol Hypertens 2006; 15(4):430–436.

(47) Skinner M, Newell E. A re-evaluation of localized hypoplasia of the primary canine as a marker of craniofacial osteopenia in European Upper Paleolithic infants. Acta Univ Carol Med (Praha) 2000; 41(1-4):41–58.

(48) Weiss E, Wetterstrom W, Nadel D et al. The broad spectrum revisited: evidence from plant remains. Proc Natl Acad Sci U S A 2004; 101(26):9551–9555.

(49) Cordain L, Eaton SB, Miller JB et al. The paradoxical nature of hunter-gatherer diets: meat-based, yet non-atherogenic. Eur J Clin Nutr 2002; 56 Suppl 1:S42–S52.

(50) Eaton SB, Eaton SB, III, Sinclair AJ et al. Dietary intake of long-chain polyunsaturated fatty acids during the paleolithic. World Rev Nutr Diet 1998; 83:12–23.

(51) Baschetti R. Paleolithic nutrition. Eur J Clin Nutr 1997; 51(10):715–716.

(52) Eaton SB, Eaton SB, III, Konner MJ. Paleolithic nutrition revisited: a twelve-year retrospective on its nature and implications. Eur J Clin Nutr 1997; 51(4):207–216.

(53) Lutz W. [The carbohydrate theory]. Wien Med Wochenschr 1994; 144(16):387–392.

(54) Jansson B. Dietary, total body, and intracellular potassium-to-sodium ratios and their influence on cancer. Cancer Detect Prev 1990; 14(5):563–565.

(55) Davis DL. Paleolithic diet, evolution, and carcinogens. Science 1987; 238(4834):1633-1634.

(56) Paleolithic nutrition. N Engl J Med 1985; 312(22):1458–1459.

(57) Eaton SB, Konner M. Paleolithic nutrition. A consideration of its nature and current implications. N Engl J Med 1985; 312(5):283–289.

(58) Strohle A, Wolters M, Hahn A. [Human nutrition in the context of evolutionary medicine]. Wien Klin Wochenschr 2009; 121(5–6):173–187.

(59) Cordain L, Eaton SB, Miller JB et al. The paradoxical nature of hunter-gatherer diets: meat-based, yet non-atherogenic. Eur J Clin Nutr 2002; 56 Suppl 1:S42–S52.

(60) Simopoulos AP. Evolutionary aspects of omega-3 fatty acids in

the food supply. Prostaglandins Leukot Essent Fatty Acids 1999; 60(5–6):421–429.

(61) Cordain L, Eaton SB, Miller JB et al. The paradoxical nature of hunter-gatherer diets: meat-based, yet non-atherogenic. Eur J Clin Nutr 2002; 56 Suppl 1:S42–S52.

(62) Goshima M, Murakami T, Nakagaki H et al. Iron, zinc, manganese and copper intakes in Japanese children aged 3 to 5 years. J Nutr Sci Vitaminol (Tokyo) 2008; 54(6):475–482.

(63) Ortigues-Marty I, Micol D, Prache S et al. Nutritional value of meat: the influence of nutrition and physical activity on vitamin B12 concentrations in ruminant tissues. Reprod Nutr Dev 2005; 45(4):453–467.

(64) Predieri G, Elviri L, Tegoni M et al. Metal chelates of 2-hydroxy-4-methylthiobutanoic acid in animal feeding. Part 2: Further characterizations, in vitro and in vivo investigations. J Inorg Biochem 2005; 99(2):627–636.

(65) Bergqvist AG, Chee CM, Lutchka L et al. Selenium deficiency associated with cardiomyopathy: a complication of the ketogenic diet. Epilepsia 2003; 44(4):618–620.

(66) Saltman PD, Strause LG. The role of trace minerals in osteoporosis. J Am Coll Nutr 1993; 12(4):384–389.

(67) Balk E, Chung M, Raman G et al. B vitamins and berries and age-related neurodegenerative disorders. Evid Rep Technol Assess (Full Rep) 2006;(134):1–161.

(68) KLENNER FR. Fatigue, normal and pathological, with special consideration of myasthenia gravis and multiple sclerosis. South Med Surg 1949; 111(9):273–277.

(69) Mount HT. Multiple sclerosis and other demyelinating diseases. Can Med Assoc J 1973; 108(11):1356.

(70) Reynolds E. Vitamin B12, folic acid, and the nervous system. Lancet Neurol 2006; 5(11):949–960.

(71) Bottiglieri T. Folate, vitamin B12, and neuropsychiatric disorders. Nutr Rev 1996; 54(12):382–390.

(72) Flicker L, Martins RN, Thomas J et al. B-vitamins reduce plasma levels of beta amyloid. Neurobiol Aging 2008; 29(2):303–305.

(73) Quadri P, Fragiacomo C, Pezzati R et al. Homocysteine and B vitamins in mild cognitive impairment and dementia. Clin Chem Lab Med 2005; 43(10):1096–1100.

(74) Rosenberg IH. B vitamins, homocysteine, and neurocognitive function. Nutr Rev 2001; 59(8 Pt 2):S69–S73.

(75) Smith AD. Prevention of dementia: a role for B vitamins? Nutr Health 2006; 18(3):225–226.

(76) Smith AD. The worldwide challenge of the dementias: a role for B vitamins and homocysteine? Food Nutr Bull 2008; 29(2 Suppl):S143–S172.

(77) Tucker KL, Qiao N, Scott T et al. High homocysteine and low B vitamins predict cognitive decline in aging men: the Veterans Affairs Normative Aging Study. Am J Clin Nutr 2005; 82(3):627–635.

(78) McCarty MF, Russell AL. Niacinamide therapy for osteoarthritis--does it inhibit nitric oxide synthase induction by interleukin 1 in chondrocytes? Med Hypotheses 1999; 53(4):350–360.

(79) Nakajima H, Yamada K, Hanafusa T et al. Elevated antibody-dependent cell-mediated cytotoxicity and its inhibition by nicotinamide in the diabetic NOD mouse. Immunol Lett 1986; 12(2-3):91–94.

(80) Yamada K, Nonaka K, Tarui S. [Prevention and therapy for diabetes associated with insulitis in non-obese diabetic mice]. Horumon To Rinsho 1982; 30(7):671–674.

(81) Yamada K, Hanafusa T, Fujino-Kurihara H et al. Nicotinamide prevents lymphocytic infiltration in submandibular glands but not the appearance of anti-salivary duct antibodies in non-obese diabetic (NOD) mice. Res Commun Chem Pathol Pharmacol 1985; 50(1):83–91.

(82) Yamada K, Nonaka K, Hanafusa T et al. Preventive and therapeutic effects of large-dose nicotinamide injections on diabetes associated with insulitis. An observation in nonobese diabetic (NOD) mice. Diabetes 1982; 31(9):749–753.

(83) Kaneko S, Wang J, Kaneko M et al. Protecting axonal degeneration by increasing nicotinamide adenine dinucleotide levels in experimental autoimmune encephalomyelitis models. J Neurosci 2006; 26(38):9794–9804.

(84) Aisen PS, Schneider LS, Sano M et al. High-dose B vitamin supplementation and cognitive decline in Alzheimer disease: a randomized controlled trial. JAMA 2008; 300(15):1774–1783.

(85) Cook S, Hess OM. Homocysteine and B vitamins. Handb Exp Pharmacol 2005;(170):325-338.

(86) Nilsson K, Gustafson L, Hultberg B. Plasma homocysteine levels and different forms of vascular disease in patients with dementia and other psychogeriatric diseases. Dement Geriatr Cogn Disord 2009; 27(1):88–95.

(87) Finsterer J. Mitochondrial disorders, cognitive impairment and dementia. J Neurol Sci 2009.

(88) Panetta J, Smith LJ, Boneh A. Effect of high-dose vitamins, coenzyme Q and high-fat diet in paediatric patients with mitochondrial diseases. J Inherit Metab Dis 2004; 27(4):487–498.

(89) Bigal ME, Krymchantowski AV, Rapoport AM. Prophylactic migraine therapy: emerging treatment options. Curr Pain Headache Rep 2004; 8(3):178–184.

(90) Magis D, Ambrosini A, Sandor P et al. A randomized double-blind placebo-controlled trial of thioctic acid in migraine prophylaxis. Headache 2007; 47(1):52–57.

(91) Tankova T, Cherninkova S, Koev D. Treatment for diabetic mononeuropathy with alpha-lipoic acid. Int J Clin Pract 2005; 59(6):645–650.

(92) Negrisanu G, Rosu M, Bolte B et al. Effects of 3-month treatment with the antioxidant alpha-lipoic acid in diabetic peripheral neuropathy. Rom J Intern Med 1999; 37(3):297–306.

(93) Tankova T, Koev D, Dakovska L. Alpha-lipoic acid in the treatment of autonomic diabetic neuropathy (controlled, randomized, open-label study). Rom J Intern Med 2004; 42(2):457-464.

(94) Calabrese V, Giuffrida Stella AM, Calvani M et al. Acetylcarnitine and cellular stress response: roles in nutritional redox homeostasis and regulation of longevity genes. J Nutr Biochem 2006; 17(2):73–88.

(95) Calabrese V, Ravagna A, Colombrita C et al. Acetylcarnitine induces heme oxygenase in rat astrocytes and protects against oxidative stress: involvement of the transcription factor Nrf2. J Neurosci Res 2005; 79(4):509–521.

(96) Pescosolido N, Imperatrice B, Karavitis P. The aging eye and the role of L-carnitine and its derivatives. Drugs R D 2008; 9 Suppl 1:3–14.

(97) Ikeda K, Negishi H, Yamori Y. Antioxidant nutrients and hypoxia/ischemia brain injury in rodents. Toxicology 2003; 189(1–2):55–61.

(98) Karuppagounder SS, Pinto JT, Xu H et al. Dietary supplementation with resveratrol reduces plaque pathology in a transgenic model of Alzheimer's disease. Neurochem Int 2009; 54(2):111–118.

(99) Sinha K, Chaudhary G, Gupta YK. Protective effect of resveratrol against oxidative stress in middle cerebral artery occlusion model of stroke in rats. Life Sci 2002; 71(6):655-665.

(100) Barger JL, Kayo T, Vann JM et al. A low dose of dietary resveratrol partially mimics caloric restriction and retards aging parameters in mice. PLoS ONE 2008; 3(6):e2264.

(101) Delmas D, Jannin B, Latruffe N. Resveratrol: preventing properties against vascular alterations and ageing. Mol Nutr Food Res

2005; 49(5):377–395.

(102) Lopez-Lluch G, Irusta PM, Navas P et al. Mitochondrial biogenesis and healthy aging. Exp Gerontol 2008; 43(9):813–819.

(103) Rossi L, Mazzitelli S, Arciello M et al. Benefits from dietary polyphenols for brain aging and Alzheimer's disease. Neurochem Res 2008; 33(12):2390–2400.

(104) Bender A, Beckers J, Schneider I et al. Creatine improves health and survival of mice. Neurobiol Aging 2008; 29(9):1404–1411.

(105) Prass K, Royl G, Lindauer U et al. Improved reperfusion and neuroprotection by creatine in a mouse model of stroke. J Cereb Blood Flow Metab 2007; 27(3):452–459.

(106) Juravleva E, Barbakadze T, Mikeladze D et al. Creatine enhances survival of glutamate-treated neuronal/glial cells, modulates Ras/NF-kappaB signaling, and increases the generation of reactive oxygen species. J Neurosci Res 2005; 79(1–2):224–230.

(107) LeWitt PA. Clinical trials of neuroprotection for Parkinson's disease. Neurology 2004; 63(7 Suppl 2):S23–S31.

(108) Rabchevsky AG, Sullivan PG, Fugaccia I et al. Creatine diet supplement for spinal cord injury: influences on functional recovery and tissue sparing in rats. J Neurotrauma 2003; 20(7):659-669.

(109) Hausmann ON, Fouad K, Wallimann T et al. Protective effects of oral creatine supplementation on spinal cord injury in rats. Spinal Cord 2002; 40(9):449–456.

(110) Brustovetsky N, Brustovetsky T, Dubinsky JM. On the mechanisms of neuroprotection by creatine and phosphocreatine. J Neurochem 2001; 76(2):425–434.

(111) Sullivan PG, Geiger JD, Mattson MP et al. Dietary supplement creatine protects against traumatic brain injury. Ann Neurol 2000; 48(5):723–729.

(112) Wilken B, Ramirez JM, Probst I et al. Anoxic ATP depletion in neonatal mice brainstem is prevented by creatine supplementation. Arch Dis Child Fetal Neonatal Ed 2000; 82(3):F224–F227.

(113) Sun-Edelstein C, Mauskop A. Role of magnesium in the pathogenesis and treatment of migraine. Expert Rev Neurother 2009; 9(3):369–379.

(114) Tepper SJ. Complementary and alternative treatments for childhood headaches. Curr Pain Headache Rep 2008; 12(5):379–383.

(115) Schurks M, Diener HC, Goadsby P. Update on the prophylaxis of migraine. Curr Treat Options Neurol 2008; 10(1):20–29.

(116) Grazzi L, Andrasik F, Usai S et al. Magnesium as a preventive

treatment for paediatric episodic tension-type headache: results at 1-year follow-up. Neurol Sci 2007; 28(3):148–150.

(117) Tramer MR, Glynn CJ. An evaluation of a single dose of magnesium to supplement analgesia after ambulatory surgery: randomized controlled trial. Anesth Analg 2007; 104(6):1374–9, table.

(118) Stillman M, Cata JP. Management of chemotherapy-induced peripheral neuropathy. Curr Pain Headache Rep 2006; 10(4):279–287.

(119) Evans RW, Taylor FR. "Natural" or alternative medications for migraine prevention. Headache 2006; 46(6):1012–1018.

(120) Woolhouse M. Migraine and tension headache—a complementary and alternative medicine approach. Aust Fam Physician 2005; 34(8):647–651.

(121) Sandor PS, Afra J. Nonpharmacologic treatment of migraine. Curr Pain Headache Rep 2005; 9(3):202–205.

(122) Altura BM, Altura BT. Tension headaches and muscle tension: is there a role for magnesium? Med Hypotheses 2001; 57(6):705–713.

(123) Gee JB, Corbett RJ, Perlman J et al. The effects of systemic magnesium sulfate infusion on brain magnesium concentrations and energy state during hypoxia-ischemia in newborn miniswine. Pediatr Res 2004; 55(1):93–100.

(124) Perlman JM. Antenatal glucocorticoid, magnesium exposure, and the prevention of brain injury of prematurity. Semin Pediatr Neurol 1998; 5(3):202-210.

(125) Gaby AR. Natural approaches to epilepsy. Altern Med Rev 2007; 12(1):9-24.

(126) El IA, Messing J, Scalia J et al. Prevention of epileptic seizures by taurine. Adv Exp Med Biol 2003; 526:515–525.

(127) Igisu H, Matsuoka M, Iryo Y. Protection of the brain by carnitine. Sangyo Eiseigaku Zasshi 1995; 37(2):75–82.

(128) Takahashi K, Azuma Y, Kobayashi S et al. Tool from traditional medicines is useful for health-medication: Bezoar Bovis and taurine. Adv Exp Med Biol 2009; 643:95–103.

(129) Yamori Y, Liu L, Mori M et al. Taurine as the nutritional factor for the longevity of the Japanese revealed by a world-wide epidemiological survey. Adv Exp Med Biol 2009; 643:13–25.

(130) Szymanski K, Winiarska K. [Taurine and its potential therapeutic application]. Postepy Hig Med Dosw (Online) 2008; 62:75–86.

(131) Freeman LM, Rush JE. Nutrition and cardiomyopathy: lessons from spontaneous animal models. Curr Heart Fail Rep 2007; 4(2):84–90.

(132) Gupta RC, Win T, Bittner S. Taurine analogues; a new class

of therapeutics: retrospect and prospects. Curr Med Chem 2005; 12(17):2021–2039.

(133) Yamori Y, Murakami S, Ikeda K et al. Fish and lifestyle-related disease prevention: experimental and epidemiological evidence for anti-atherogenic potential of taurine. Clin Exp Pharmacol Physiol 2004; 31 Suppl 2:S20–S23

(134) Kingston R, Kelly CJ, Murray P. The therapeutic role of taurine in ischaemia-reperfusion injury. Curr Pharm Des 2004; 10(19):2401–2410.

(135) Pathirana C, Grimble RF. Taurine and serine supplementation modulates the metabolic response to tumor necrosis factor alpha in rats fed a low protein diet. J Nutr 1992; 122(7):1369–1375.

(136) Lakhan SE, Vieira KF. Nutritional therapies for mental disorders. Nutr J 2008; 7:2.

(137) Parcell S. Sulfur in human nutrition and applications in medicine. Altern Med Rev 2002; 7(1):22–44.

(138) Moss RL, Haynes AL, Pastuszyn A et al. Methionine infusion reproduces liver injury of parenteral nutrition cholestasis. Pediatr Res 1999; 45(5 Pt 1):664–668.

(139) Nencini C, Giorgi G, Micheli L. Protective effect of silymarin on oxidative stress in rat brain. Phytomedicine 2007; 14(2–3):129–135.

(140) Toklu HZ, Tunali AT, Velioglu-Ogunc A et al. Silymarin, the antioxidant component of Silybum marianum, prevents sepsis-induced acute lung and brain injury. J Surg Res 2008; 145(2):214–222.

(141) Nirala SK, Bhadauria M. Propolis reverses acetaminophen induced acute hepatorenal alterations: a biochemical and histopathological approach. Arch Pharm Res 2008; 31(4):451–461.

(142) Rastogi R, Srivastava AK, Rastogi AK. Long term effect of aflatoxin B(1) on lipid peroxidation in rat liver and kidney: effect of picroliv and silymarin. Phytother Res 2001; 15(4):307–310.

(143) Duthie SJ, Johnson W, Dobson VL. The effect of dietary flavonoids on DNA damage (strand breaks and oxidised pyrimdines) and growth in human cells. Mutat Res 1997; 390(1–2):141–151.

(144) Duvoix A, Delhalle S, Blasius R et al. Effect of chemopreventive agents on glutathione S-transferase P1-1 gene expression mechanisms via activating protein 1 and nuclear factor kappaB inhibition. Biochem Pharmacol 2004; 68(6):1101–1111.

(145) Lieber CS. Alcoholic liver disease: new insights in pathogenesis lead to new treatments. J Hepatol 2000; 32(1 Suppl):113–128.

(146) Mantena SK, Katiyar SK. Grape seed proanthocyanidins inhibit UV-radiation-induced oxidative stress and activation of MAPK and NF-

kappaB signaling in human epidermal keratinocytes. Free Radic Biol Med 2006; 40(9):1603–1614.

(147) Wellington K, Jarvis B. Silymarin: a review of its clinical properties in the management of hepatic disorders. BioDrugs 2001; 15(7):465–489.

(148) Sharma D, Sethi P, Hussain E et al. Curcumin counteracts the aluminium-induced ageing-related alterations in oxidative stress, Na(+), K (+) ATPase and protein kinase C in adult and old rat brain regions. Biogerontology 2008.

(149) Rowe MK, Chuang DM. Lithium neuroprotection: molecular mechanisms and clinical implications. Expert Rev Mol Med 2004; 6(21):1–18.

(150) Pari L, Murugan P. Tetrahydrocurcumin prevents brain lipid peroxidation in streptozotocin-induced diabetic rats. J Med Food 2007; 10(2):323–329.

(151) El-Demerdash FM, Yousef MI, Radwan FM. Ameliorating effect of curcumin on sodium arsenite-induced oxidative damage and lipid peroxidation in different rat organs. Food Chem Toxicol 2009; 47(1):249–254.

(152) Batcioglu K, Karagozler AA, Ozturk IC et al. Comparison of chemopreventive effects of Vitamin E plus selenium versus melatonin in 7,12-dimethylbenz(a)anthracene-induced mouse brain damage. Cancer Detect Prev 2005; 29(1):54–58.

(153) Simoni J, Simoni G, Garcia EL et al. Protective effect of selenium on hemoglobin mediated lipid peroxidation in vivo. Artif Cells Blood Substit Immobil Biotechnol 1995; 23(4):469–486.

(154) Borek C. Antioxidant health effects of aged garlic extract. J Nutr 2001; 131(3s):1010S-1015S.

(155) Cheng W, Fu YX, Porres JM et al. Selenium-dependent cellular glutathione peroxidase protects mice against a pro-oxidant-induced oxidation of NADPH, NADH, lipids, and protein. FASEB J 1999; 13(11):1467–1475.

(156) Egashira N, Hayakawa K, Mishima K et al. Neuroprotective effect of gamma-glutamylethylamide (theanine) on cerebral infarction in mice. Neurosci Lett 2004; 363(1):58-61.

(157) Kimura R, Murata T. Effect of theanine on norepinephrine and serotonin levels in rat brain. Chem Pharm Bull (Tokyo) 1986; 34(7):3053–3057.

(158) Yokogoshi H, Kobayashi M, Mochizuki M et al. Effect of theanine, r-glutamylethylamide, on brain monoamines and striatal dopamine release

in conscious rats. Neurochem Res 1998; 23(5):667–673.

(159) Cho HS, Kim S, Lee SY et al. Protective effect of the green tea component, L-theanine on environmental toxins-induced neuronal cell death. Neurotoxicology 2008; 29(4):656-662.

(160) Nathan PJ, Lu K, Gray M et al. The neuropharmacology of L-theanine(N-ethyl-L-glutamine): a possible neuroprotective and cognitive enhancing agent. J Herb Pharmacother 2006; 6(2):21-30.

(161) Yamada T, Terashima T, Okubo T et al. Effects of theanine, r-glutamylethylamide, on neurotransmitter release and its relationship with glutamic acid neurotransmission. Nutr Neurosci 2005; 8(4):219–226.

(162) Yamada T, Terashima T, Kawano S et al. Theanine, gamma-glutamylethylamide, a unique amino acid in tea leaves, modulates neurotransmitter concentrations in the brain striatum interstitium in conscious rats. Amino Acids 2009; 36(1):21–27.

(163) Yamada T, Terashima T, Wada K et al. Theanine, r-glutamylethylamide, increases neurotransmission concentrations and neurotrophin mRNA levels in the brain during lactation. Life Sci 2007; 81(16):1247–1255.

(164) Yokogoshi H, Kobayashi M, Mochizuki M et al. Effect of theanine, r-glutamylethylamide, on brain monoamines and striatal dopamine release in conscious rats. Neurochem Res 1998; 23(5):667–673.

(165) Yokogoshi H, Terashima T. Effect of theanine, r-glutamylethylamide, on brain monoamines, striatal dopamine release and some kinds of behavior in rats. Nutrition 2000; 16(9):776-777.

(166) Meeusen R. Exercise and the brain: insight in new therapeutic modalities. Ann Transplant 2005; 10(4):49–51.

(167) Sarbadhikari SN, Saha AK. Moderate exercise and chronic stress produce counteractive effects on different areas of the brain by acting through various neurotransmitter receptor subtypes: a hypothesis. Theor Biol Med Model 2006; 3:33.

(168) Mouyis M, Ostor AJ, Crisp AJ et al. Hypovitaminosis D among rheumatology outpatients in clinical practice. Rheumatology (Oxford) 2008; 47(9):1348–1351.

(169) Schwalfenberg G. Improvement of chronic back pain or failed back surgery with vitamin D repletion: a case series. J Am Board Fam Med 2009; 22(1):69–74.

(170) Bartley J. Prevalence of vitamin D deficiency among patients attending a multidisciplinary tertiary pain clinic. N Z Med J 2008; 121(1286):57–62.

(171) Berk M, Jacka FN, Williams LJ et al. Is this D vitamin to worry about? Vitamin D insufficiency in an inpatient sample. Aust N Z J Psychiatry 2008; 42(10):874–878.

(172) Vitamin D supplement in early childhood and risk for Type I (insulin-dependent) diabetes mellitus. The EURODIAB Substudy 2 Study Group. Diabetologia 1999; 42(1):51–54.

(173) Franchimont N, Canalis E. Management of glucocorticoid induced osteoporosis in premenopausal women with autoimmune disease. Autoimmun Rev 2003; 2(4):224–228.

(174) Gaby AR. Natural remedies for scleroderma. Altern Med Rev 2006; 11(3):188–195.

(175) Garton M, Reid I, Loveridge N et al. Bone mineral density and metabolism in premenopausal women taking L-thyroxine replacement therapy. Clin Endocrinol (Oxf) 1994; 41(6):747–755.

(176) Norval M. The mechanisms and consequences of ultraviolet-induced immunosuppression. Prog Biophys Mol Biol 2006; 92(1):108–118.

(177) Patavino T, Brady DM. Natural medicine and nutritional therapy as an alternative treatment in systemic lupus erythematosus. Altern Med Rev 2001; 6(5):460–471.

(178) Freedman DM, Fuhrman B, Graubard BI et al. Vitamin D and cancer mortality. Cancer Epidemiol Biomarkers Prev 2009; 18(1):359–360.

(179) Kilkkinen A, Knekt P, Heliovaara M et al. Vitamin D status and the risk of lung cancer: a cohort study in Finland. Cancer Epidemiol Biomarkers Prev 2008; 17(11):3274–3278.

(180) McCombie AM, Mason RS, Damian DL. Vitamin D deficiency in Sydney skin cancer patients. Med J Aust 2009; 190(2):102.

(181) Mohr SB. A brief history of vitamin d and cancer prevention. Ann Epidemiol 2009; 19(2):79–83.

(182) Berk M, Sanders KM, Pasco JA et al. Vitamin D deficiency may play a role in depression. Med Hypotheses 2007; 69(6):1316–1319.

(183) Young SN. Has the time come for clinical trials on the antidepressant effect of vitamin D? J Psychiatry Neurosci 2009; 34(1):3.

(184) Tai K, Need AG, Horowitz M et al. Glucose tolerance and vitamin D: effects of treating vitamin D deficiency. Nutrition 2008; 24(10):950–956.

(185) Findling RL, McNamara NK, O'Riordan MA et al. An open-label pilot study of St. John's wort in juvenile depression. J Am Acad Child Adolesc Psychiatry 2003; 42(8):908–914.

(186) Kasper S. Hypericum perforatum—a review of clinical studies. Pharmacopsychiatry 2001; 34 Suppl 1:S51–S55.

(187) Whiskey E, Werneke U, Taylor D. A systematic review and meta-analysis of Hypericum perforatum in depression: a comprehensive clinical review. Int Clin Psychopharmacol 2001; 16(5):239–252.

(188) Cotman CW, Berchtold NC. Exercise: a behavioral intervention to enhance brain health and plasticity. Trends Neurosci 2002; 25(6):295–301.

(189) Albeck DS, Beck KD, Kung LH et al. Leverpress escape/avoidance training increases neurotrophin levels in rat brain. Integr Physiol Behav Sci 2005; 40(1):28–34.

(190) Exercising to keep aging at bay. Nat Neurosci 2007; 10(3):263.

(191) Small GW, Silverman DH, Siddarth P et al. Effects of a 14-day healthy longevity lifestyle program on cognition and brain function. Am J Geriatr Psychiatry 2006; 14(6):538–545.

(192) Luo Y. Ginkgo biloba neuroprotection: Therapeutic implications in Alzheimer's disease. J Alzheimers Dis 2001; 3(4):401–407.

(193) Kidd PM. Neurodegeneration from mitochondrial insufficiency: nutrients, stem cells, growth factors, and prospects for brain rebuilding using integrative management. Altern Med Rev 2005; 10(4):268–293.

(194) Molyneux SL, Young JM, Florkowski CM et al. Coenzyme q10: is there a clinical role and a case for measurement? Clin Biochem Rev 2008; 29(2):71–82.

(195) Beal MF. Coenzyme Q10 as a possible treatment for neurodegenerative diseases. Free Radic Res 2002; 36(4):455-460.

(196) Kidd PM. Neurodegeneration from mitochondrial insufficiency: nutrients, stem cells, growth factors, and prospects for brain rebuilding using integrative management. Altern Med Rev 2005; 10(4):268–293.

(197) Chuang DM. Neuroprotective and neurotrophic actions of the mood stabilizer lithium: can it be used to treat neurodegenerative diseases? Crit Rev Neurobiol 2004; 16(1-2):83–90.

(198) Chuang DM. The antiapoptotic actions of mood stabilizers: molecular mechanisms and therapeutic potentials. Ann N Y Acad Sci 2005; 1053:195–204.

(199) Hashimoto R, Fujimaki K, Jeong MR et al. [Neuroprotective actions of lithium]. Seishin Shinkeigaku Zasshi 2003; 105(1):81–86.

(200) De SP, Axtell RC, Raman C et al. Lithium prevents and ameliorates experimental autoimmune encephalomyelitis. J Immunol 2008; 181(1):338–345.

(201) Compher C, Badellino KO. Obesity and inflammation: lessons

from bariatric surgery. JPEN J Parenter Enteral Nutr 2008; 32(6):645–647.

(202) de LC, Olefsky JM. Inflammation and insulin resistance. FEBS Lett 2008; 582(1):97–105.

(203) Fornoni A, Ijaz A, Tejada T et al. Role of inflammation in diabetic nephropathy. Curr Diabetes Rev 2008; 4(1):10–17.

(204) Guandalini S, Setty M. Celiac disease. Curr Opin Gastroenterol 2008; 24(6):707–712.

(205) Catassi C, Fasano A. Celiac disease. Curr Opin Gastroenterol 2008; 24(6):687–691.

(206) Ravikumara M, Tuthill DP, Jenkins HR. The changing clinical presentation of coeliac disease. Arch Dis Child 2006; 91(12):969–971.

(207) Addolorato G, Di GD, De RG et al. Regional cerebral hypoperfusion in patients with celiac disease. Am J Med 2004; 116(5):312–317.

(208) Serratrice J, Disdier P, Kaladjian A et al. [Psychosis revealing a silent celiac disease in a young women with trisomy 21]. Presse Med 2002; 31(33):1551–1553.

(209) Yucel B, Ozbey N, Demir K et al. Eating disorders and celiac disease: a case report. Int J Eat Disord 2006; 39(6):530–532.

(210) Eberman LE, Cleary MA. Celiac disease in an elite female collegiate volleyball athlete: a case report. J Athl Train 2005; 40(4):360–364.

(211) Csak T, Folhoffer A, Horvath A et al. Holmes-Adie syndrome, autoimmune hepatitis and celiac disease: a case report. World J Gastroenterol 2006; 12(9):1485–1487.

(212) Goodman BP, Mistry DH, Pasha SF et al. Copper deficiency myeloneuropathy due to occult celiac disease. Neurologist 2009; 15(6):355–356.

(213) Poloni N, Vender S, Bolla E et al. Gluten encephalopathy with psychiatric onset: case report. Clin Pract Epidemol Ment Health 2009; 5:16.

(214) Simonati A, Battistella PA, Guariso G et al. Coeliac disease associated with peripheral neuropathy in a child: a case report. Neuropediatrics 1998; 29(3):155–158.

(215) Brown KJ, Jewells V, Herfarth H et al. White Matter Lesions Suggestive of Amyotrophic Lateral Sclerosis Attributed to Celiac Disease. AJNR Am J Neuroradiol 2009.\

(216)   Cartalat-Carel S, Pradat PF, Carpentier A et al. [Chronic meningitis before diagnosis of celiac disease]. Rev Neurol (Paris) 2002;

158(4):467–469.

(217) Hsu CL, Lin CY, Chen CL et al. The effects of a gluten and casein-free diet in children with autism: a case report. Chang Gung Med J 2009; 32(4):459–465.

(218) Maes M, Twisk FN. Chronic fatigue syndrome: la bete noire of the Belgian health care system. Neuro Endocrinol Lett 2009; 30(3):300–311.

(219) Terjung B, Spengler U. Atypical p-ANCA in PSC and AIH: a hint toward a "leaky gut"? Clin Rev Allergy Immunol 2009; 36(1):40–51.

(220) Russo AF. Anti-metallothionein IgG and levels of metallothionein in autistic families. Swiss Med Wkly 2008; 138(5–6):70–77.

(221) Maes M, Coucke F, Leunis JC. Normalization of the increased translocation of endotoxin from gram negative enterobacteria (leaky gut) is accompanied by a remission of chronic fatigue syndrome. Neuro Endocrinol Lett 2007; 28(6):739–744.

(222) Maes M. Inflammatory and oxidative and nitrosative stress pathways underpinning chronic fatigue, somatization and psychosomatic symptoms. Curr Opin Psychiatry 2009; 22(1):75–83.

(223) Maes M, Leunis JC. Normalization of leaky gut in chronic fatigue syndrome (CFS) is accompanied by a clinical improvement: effects of age, duration of illness and the translocation of LPS from gram-negative bacteria. Neuro Endocrinol Lett 2008; 29(6):902–910.

(224) Maes M, Kubera M, Leunis JC. The gut-brain barrier in major depression: intestinal mucosal dysfunction with an increased translocation of LPS from gram negative enterobacteria (leaky gut) plays a role in the inflammatory pathophysiology of depression. Neuro Endocrinol Lett 2008; 29(1):117–124.

(225) Ukena SN, Singh A, Dringenberg U et al. Probiotic Escherichia coli Nissle 1917 inhibits leaky gut by enhancing mucosal integrity. PLoS ONE 2007; 2(12):e1308.

(226) Maes M. The cytokine hypothesis of depression: inflammation, oxidative & nitrosative stress (IO&NS) and leaky gut as new targets for adjunctive treatments in depression. Neuro Endocrinol Lett 2008; 29(3):287–291.

(227) Carson R. Anv ed. Mariner Books, 2002

(228) Barraj LM, Scrafford CG, Eaton WC et al. Arsenic levels in wipe samples collected from play structures constructed with CCA-treated wood: impact on exposure estimates. Sci Total Environ 2009; 407(8):2586–2592.

(229) Barraj LM, Tsuji JS, Scrafford CG. The SHEDS-Wood model:

incorporation of observational data to estimate exposure to arsenic for children playing on CCA-treated wood structures. Environ Health Perspect 2007; 115(5):781–786.

(230) Kwon E, Zhang H, Wang Z et al. Arsenic on the hands of children after playing in playgrounds. Environ Health Perspect 2004; 112(14):1375–1380.

(231) Pike-Paris A. Arsenic in a child's world. Pediatr Nurs 2004; 30(3):215–218.

(232) Barr DB, Bishop A, Needham LL. Concentrations of xenobiotic chemicals in the maternal-fetal unit. Reprod Toxicol 2007; 23(3):260–266.

(233) Byczkowski JZ, Gearhart JM, Fisher JW. "Occupational" exposure of infants to toxic chemicals via breast milk. Nutrition 1994; 10(1):43–48.

(234) Crinnion WJ. Maternal levels of xenobiotics that affect fetal development and childhood health. Altern Med Rev 2009; 14(3):212–222.

(235) Giacoia GP, Catz C, Yaffe SJ. Environmental hazards in milk and infant nutrition. Clin Obstet Gynecol 1983; 26(2):458–466.

(236) Howard CR, Lawrence RA. Xenobiotics and breastfeeding. Pediatr Clin North Am 2001; 48(2):485–504.

(237) Meyer I, Heinrich J, Lippold U. Factors affecting lead and cadmium levels in house dust in industrial areas of eastern Germany. Sci Total Environ 1999; 234(1–3):25–36.

(238) Chang LW. The neurotoxicology and pathology of organomercury, organolead, and organotin. J Toxicol Sci 1990; 15 Suppl 4:125–151.

(239) Mutter J, Naumann J, Schneider R et al. [Mercury and Alzheimer's disease]. Fortschr Neurol Psychiatr 2007; 75(9):528–538.

(240) Mutter J, Naumann J, Guethlin C. Comments on the article "the toxicology of mercury and its chemical compounds" by Clarkson and Magos (2006). Crit Rev Toxicol 2007; 37(6):537-549.

(241) Mutter J, Naumann J, Sadaghiani C et al. Amalgam studies: disregarding basic principles of mercury toxicity. Int J Hyg Environ Health 2004; 207(4):391–397.

(242)   Anway MD, Skinner MK. Epigenetic transgenerational actions of endocrine disruptors. Endocrinology 2006; 147(6 Suppl):S43–S49.

(243)   Skinner MK, Anway MD. Seminiferous cord formation and germ-cell programming: epigenetic transgenerational actions of endocrine disruptors. Ann N Y Acad Sci 2005; 1061:18–32.

(244) Hombach-Klonisch S, Pocar P, Kauffold J et al. Dioxin exerts anti-estrogenic actions in a novel dioxin-responsive telomerase-immortalized epithelial cell line of the porcine oviduct (TERT-OPEC). Toxicol Sci 2006; 90(2):519–528.

(245) Anway MD, Cupp AS, Uzumcu M et al. Epigenetic transgenerational actions of endocrine disruptors and male fertility. Science 2005; 308(5727):1466–1469.

(246) Trasande L, Schechter CB, Haynes KA et al. Mental retardation and prenatal methylmercury toxicity. Am J Ind Med 2006; 49(3):153–158.

(247) Sanfeliu C, Sebastia J, Cristofol R et al. Neurotoxicity of organomercurial compounds. Neurotox Res 2003; 5(4):283–305.

(248) Patrick L. Mercury toxicity and antioxidants: Part 1: role of glutathione and alpha-lipoic acid in the treatment of mercury toxicity. Altern Med Rev 2002; 7(6):456–471.

(249) Rodier PM. Developing brain as a target of toxicity. Environ Health Perspect 1995; 103 Suppl 6:73–76.

(250) Valk J, van der Knaap MS. Toxic encephalopathy. AJNR Am J Neuroradiol 1992; 13(2):747-760.

(251) Aminzadeh KK, Etminan M. Dental amalgam and multiple sclerosis: a systematic review and meta-analysis. J Public Health Dent 2007; 67(1):64–66.

(252) Bangsi D, Ghadirian P, Ducic S et al. Dental amalgam and multiple sclerosis: a case-control study in Montreal, Canada. Int J Epidemiol 1998; 27(4):667–671.

(253) Casetta I, Invernizzi M, Granieri E. Multiple sclerosis and dental amalgam: case-control study in Ferrara, Italy. Neuroepidemiology 2001; 20(2):134–137.

(254) Clausen J. Mercury and multiple sclerosis. Acta Neurol Scand 1993; 87(6):461-464.

(255) deShazer DO. The mercury-multiple sclerosis connection. J Colo Dent Assoc 1985; 63(4):4.

(256) Fung YK, Meade AG, Rack EP et al. Brain mercury in neurodegenerative disorders. J Toxicol Clin Toxicol 1997; 35(1):49–54.

(257) Eggleston DW, Nylander M. Correlation of dental amalgam with mercury in brain tissue. J Prosthet Dent 1987; 58(6):704–707.

(258) Feng Q, Keshtgarpour M, Pelleymounter LL et al. Human S-adenosylhomocysteine hydrolase: common gene sequence variation and functional genomic characterization. J Neurochem 2009; 110(6):1806–1817.

(259) Hernandez A, Xamena N, Surralles J et al. Role of the Met(287) Thr polymorphism in the AS3MT gene on the metabolic arsenic profile. Mutat Res 2008; 637(1-2):80–92.

(260) Singh C, Ahmad I, Kumar A. Pesticides and metals induced Parkinson's disease: involvement of free radicals and oxidative stress. Cell Mol Biol (Noisy-le-grand) 2007; 53(5):19-28.

(261) Brown TP, Rumsby PC, Capleton AC et al. Pesticides and Parkinson's disease—is there a link? Environ Health Perspect 2006; 114(2):156–164.

(262) Butterfield PG, Valanis BG, Spencer PS et al. Environmental antecedents of young-onset Parkinson's disease. Neurology 1993; 43(6):1150–1158.

(263) Caboni P, Sherer TB, Zhang N et al. Rotenone, deguelin, their metabolites, and the rat model of Parkinson's disease. Chem Res Toxicol 2004; 17(11):1540–1548.

(264) Klintworth H, Newhouse K, Li T et al. Activation of c-Jun N-terminal protein kinase is a common mechanism underlying paraquat- and rotenone-induced dopaminergic cell apoptosis. Toxicol Sci 2007; 97(1):149–162.

(265) Montgomery EB, Jr. Heavy metals and the etiology of Parkinson's disease and other movement disorders. Toxicology 1995; 97(1–3):3–9.

(266) Roth JA, Garrick MD. Iron interactions and other biological reactions mediating the physiological and toxic actions of manganese. Biochem Pharmacol 2003; 66(1):1–13.

(267) Ladd-Acosta C, Pevsner J, Sabunciyan S et al. DNA methylation signatures within the human brain. Am J Hum Genet 2007; 81(6):1304–1315.

(268) Bensemain F, Hot D, Ferreira S et al. Evidence for induction of the ornithine transcarbamylase expression in Alzheimer's disease. Mol Psychiatry 2009; 14(1):106–116.

(269) Ruf N, Bahring S, Galetzka D et al. Sequence-based bioinformatic prediction and QUASEP identify genomic imprinting of the KCNK9 potassium channel gene in mouse and human. Hum Mol Genet 2007; 16(21):2591–2599.

(270) Iwamoto K, Bundo M, Yamada K et al. A family-based and case-control association study of SOX10 in schizophrenia. Am J Med Genet B Neuropsychiatr Genet 2006; 141B(5):477–481.

(271) Dempster EL, Mill J, Craig IW et al. The quantification of COMT mRNA in post mortem cerebellum tissue: diagnosis, genotype,

methylation and expression. BMC Med Genet 2006; 7:10.

(272) Murphy BC, O'Reilly RL, Singh SM. Site-specific cytosine methylation in S-COMT promoter in 31 brain regions with implications for studies involving schizophrenia. Am J Med Genet B Neuropsychiatr Genet 2005; 133B(1):37–42.

(273) Maegawa S, Itaba N, Otsuka S et al. Coordinate downregulation of a novel imprinted transcript ITUP1 with PEG3 in glioma cell lines. DNA Res 2004; 11(1):37–49.

(274) Ronai Z, Witt H, Rickards O et al. A common African polymorphism abolishes tyrosine sulfation of human anionic trypsinogen (PRSS2). Biochem J 2009; 418(1):155–161.

(275) van der Deure WM, Friesema EC, de Jong FJ et al. Organic anion transporter 1B1: an important factor in hepatic thyroid hormone and estrogen transport and metabolism. Endocrinology 2008; 149(9):4695–4701.

(276) Ung D, Nagar S. Variable sulfation of dietary polyphenols by recombinant human sulfotransferase (SULT) 1A1 genetic variants and SULT1E1. Drug Metab Dispos 2007; 35(5):740–746.

(277) Wilborn TW, Lang NP, Smith M et al. Association of SULT2A1 allelic variants with plasma adrenal androgens and prostate cancer in African American men. J Steroid Biochem Mol Biol 2006; 99(4–5):209–214.

(278) Nowell S, Falany CN. Pharmacogenetics of human cytosolic sulfotransferases. Oncogene 2006; 25(11):1673-1678.

(279) Adjei AA, Thomae BA, Prondzinski JL et al. Human estrogen sulfotransferase (SULT1E1) pharmacogenomics: gene resequencing and functional genomics. Br J Pharmacol 2003; 139(8):1373–1382.

(280) Ikeda T, Mabuchi A, Fukuda A et al. Identification of sequence polymorphisms in two sulfation-related genes, PAPSS2 and SLC26A2, and an association analysis with knee osteoarthritis. J Hum Genet 2001; 46(9):538–543.

(281) Giovannoni G. Management of secondary-progressive multiple sclerosis. CNS Drugs 2004; 18(10):653–669.

(282) Rovaris M, Confavreux C, Furlan R et al. Secondary progressive multiple sclerosis: current knowledge and future challenges. Lancet Neurol 2006; 5(4):343–354.

(283) Tremlett H, Zhao Y, Devonshire V. Natural history of secondary-progressive multiple sclerosis. Mult Scler 2008.

(284) Fox EJ. Management of worsening multiple sclerosis with mitoxantrone: a review. Clin Ther 2006; 28(4):461–474.

(285) Rice GP. The natural history of secondary progressive multiple sclerosis: observations from the London study group. Mult Scler 2002; 8(1):81–82.

(286) Tubridy N, Coles AJ, Molyneux P et al. Secondary progressive multiple sclerosis: the relationship between short-term MRI activity and clinical features. Brain 1998; 121 (Pt 2):225-231.

(287) Patti F, Ciancio MR, Cacopardo M et al. Effects of a short outpatient rehabilitation treatment on disability of multiple sclerosis patients—a randomised controlled trial. J Neurol 2003; 250(7):861-866.

(288) Thomaides TN, Zoukos Y, Chaudhuri KR et al. Physiological assessment of aspects of autonomic function in patients with secondary progressive multiple sclerosis. J Neurol 1993; 240(3):139–143.

(289) Daly JJ, Roenigk K, Holcomb J et al. A randomized controlled trial of functional neuromuscular stimulation in chronic stroke subjects. Stroke 2006; 37(1):172–178.

(290) Lake DA. Neuromuscular electrical stimulation. An overview and its application in the treatment of sports injuries. Sports Med 1992; 13(5):320–336.

(291) Krause P, Szecsi J, Straube A. FES cycling reduces spastic muscle tone in a patient with multiple sclerosis. NeuroRehabilitation 2007; 22(4):335–337.

(292)   McClurg D, Ashe RG, Lowe-Strong AS. Neuromuscular electrical stimulation and the treatment of lower urinary tract dysfunction in multiple sclerosis—a double blind, placebo controlled, randomised clinical trial. Neurourol Urodyn 2008; 27(3):231–237.

(293) Cotman CW, Berchtold NC, Christie LA. Exercise builds brain health: key roles of growth factor cascades and inflammation. Trends Neurosci 2007; 30(9):464–472.

(294) Busiguina S, Fernandez AM, Barrios V et al. Neurodegeneration is associated to changes in serum insulin-like growth factors. Neurobiol Dis 2000; 7(6 Pt B):657–665.

(295) Carro E, Trejo JL, Busiguina S et al. Circulating insulin-like growth factor I mediates the protective effects of physical exercise against brain insults of different etiology and anatomy. J Neurosci 2001; 21(15):5678–5684.

(296)   Facchinetti F, Dawson VL, Dawson TM. Free radicals as mediators of neuronal injury. Cell Mol Neurobiol 1998; 18(6):667–682.

(297)   Gironi M, Furlan R, Rovaris M et al. Beta endorphin concentrations in PBMC of patients with different clinical phenotypes of multiple sclerosis. J Neurol Neurosurg Psychiatry 2003; 74(4):495–497.

(298) Lipids and multiple sclerosis. Lancet 1990; 336(8706):25–26.

(299) Calder PC. n-3 polyunsaturated fatty acids and cytokine production in health and disease. Ann Nutr Metab 1997; 41(4):203–234

(300) Hayes CE, Cantorna MT, Deluca HF. Vitamin D and multiple sclerosis. Proc Soc Exp Biol Med 1997; 216(1):21–27.

(301) Nordvik I, Myhr KM, Nyland H et al. Effect of dietary advice and n-3 supplementation in newly diagnosed MS patients. Acta Neurol Scand 2000; 102(3):143–149.

(302) Simopoulos AP. Omega-3 fatty acids in inflammation and autoimmune diseases. J Am Coll Nutr 2002; 21(6):495–505.

(303) Weinstock-Guttman B, Baier M, Park Y et al. Low fat dietary intervention with omega-3 fatty acid supplementation in multiple sclerosis patients. Prostaglandins Leukot Essent Fatty Acids 2005; 73(5):397–404

(304) Cantorna MT, Mahon BD. Mounting evidence for vitamin D as an environmental factor affecting autoimmune disease prevalence. Exp Biol Med (Maywood) 2004; 229(11):1136–1142.

(305) Cantorna MT. Vitamin D and its role in immunology: multiple sclerosis, and inflammatory bowel disease. Prog Biophys Mol Biol 2006; 92(1):60–64.

(306) Hayes CE, Cantorna MT, Deluca HF. Vitamin D and multiple sclerosis. Proc Soc Exp Biol Med 1997; 216(1):21–27.

(307) Holick MF. Evolution and function of vitamin D. Recent Results Cancer Res 2003; 164:3-28.

(308) Kampman MT, Brustad M. Vitamin D: A Candidate for the Environmental Effect in Multiple Sclerosis - Observations from Norway. Neuroepidemiology 2008; 30(3):140–146.

(309) Miller A, Korem M, Almog R et al. Vitamin B12, demyelination, remyelination and repair in multiple sclerosis. J Neurol Sci 2005; 233(1-2):93–97.

(310) Kakar S, Nehra V, Murray JA et al. Significance of intraepithelial lymphocytosis in small bowel biopsy samples with normal mucosal architecture. Am J Gastroenterol 2003; 98(9):2027–2033.

(311) Volta U, De GR, Petrolini N et al. Clinical findings and anti-neuronal antibodies in coeliac disease with neurological disorders. Scand J Gastroenterol 2002; 37(11):1276–1281.

(312) Hewson DC. Is there a role for gluten-free diets in multiple sclerosis? Hum Nutr Appl Nutr 1984; 38(6):417–420.

(313) Hunter AL, Rees BW, Jones LT. Gluten antibodies in patients with multiple sclerosis. Hum Nutr Appl Nutr 1984; 38(2):142–143.

(314) Jones PE, Pallis C, Peters TJ. Morphological and biochemical

findings in jejunal biopsies from patients with multiple sclerosis. J Neurol Neurosurg Psychiatry 1979; 42(5):402–406.

(315) Patti F, Ciancio MR, Cacopardo M et al. Effects of a short outpatient rehabilitation treatment on disability of multiple sclerosis patients—a randomised controlled trial. J Neurol 2003; 250(7):861–866.

(316) Beal MF. Bioenergetic approaches for neuroprotection in Parkinson's disease. Ann Neurol 2003; 53 Suppl 3:S39–S47.

(317) Brustovetsky N, Brustovetsky T, Dubinsky JM. On the mechanisms of neuroprotection by creatine and phosphocreatine. J Neurochem 2001; 76(2):425–434.

(318) Chen RW, Chuang DM. Long term lithium treatment suppresses p53 and Bax expression but increases Bcl-2 expression. A prominent role in neuroprotection against excitotoxicity. J Biol Chem 1999; 274(10):6039–6042.

(319) Kolker S, Ahlemeyer B, Krieglstein J et al. Contribution of reactive oxygen species to 3-hydroxyglutarate neurotoxicity in primary neuronal cultures from chick embryo telencephalons. Pediatr Res 2001; 50(1):76–82.

(320) Malcon C, Kaddurah-Daouk R, Beal MF. Neuroprotective effects of creatine administration against NMDA and malonate toxicity. Brain Res 2000; 860(1-2):195–198.

(321) Qi X, Lewin AS, Sun L et al. Suppression of mitochondrial oxidative stress provides long-term neuroprotection in experimental optic neuritis. Invest Ophthalmol Vis Sci 2007; 48(2):681–691.

(322) Tseng WP, Lin-Shiau SY. Long-term lithium treatment prevents neurotoxic effects of beta-bungarotoxin in primary cultured neurons. J Neurosci Res 2002; 69(5):633–641.

(323) Qi X, Lewin AS, Sun L et al. Suppression of mitochondrial oxidative stress provides long-term neuroprotection in experimental optic neuritis. Invest Ophthalmol Vis Sci 2007; 48(2):681–691.

(324) Dhib-Jalbut S, Arnold DL, Cleveland DW et al. Neurodegeneration and neuroprotection in multiple sclerosis and other neurodegenerative diseases. J Neuroimmunol 2006; 176(1–2):198-215.

(325) Gonsette RE. Oxidative stress and excitotoxicity: a therapeutic issue in multiple sclerosis? Mult Scler 2008; 14(1):22–34.

(326) Hague T, Andrews PL, Barker J et al. Dietary chelators as antioxidant enzyme mimetics: implications for dietary intervention in neurodegenerative diseases. Behav Pharmacol 2006; 17(5–6):425–430.

(327) Juurlink BH. Therapeutic potential of dietary phase 2 enzyme inducers in ameliorating diseases that have an underlying inflammatory

component. Can J Physiol Pharmacol 2001; 79(3):266–282.

(328) Mohamed AA, Avila JG, Schultke E et al. Amelioration of experimental allergic encephalitis (EAE) through phase 2 enzyme induction. Biomed Sci Instrum 2002; 38:9–13.

(329) Payne A. Nutrition and diet in the clinical management of multiple sclerosis. J Hum Nutr Diet 2001; 14(5):349–357.

(330) Syburra C, Passi S. Oxidative stress in patients with multiple sclerosis. Ukr Biokhim Zh 1999; 71(3):112–115.

(331) van Meeteren ME, Teunissen CE, Dijkstra CD et al. Antioxidants and polyunsaturated fatty acids in multiple sclerosis. Eur J Clin Nutr 2005; 59(12):1347–1361.

(332)   Sarchielli P, Greco L, Floridi A et al. Excitatory amino acids and multiple sclerosis: evidence from cerebrospinal fluid. Arch Neurol 2003; 60(8):1082–1088.

(333) Vercellino M, Merola A, Piacentino C et al. Altered glutamate reuptake in relapsing-remitting and secondary progressive multiple sclerosis cortex: correlation with microglia infiltration, demyelination, and neuronal and synaptic damage. J Neuropathol Exp Neurol 2007; 66(8):732–739.

(334) Vercellino M, Merola A, Piacentino C et al. Altered glutamate reuptake in relapsing-remitting and secondary progressive multiple sclerosis cortex: correlation with microglia infiltration, demyelination, and neuronal and synaptic damage. J Neuropathol Exp Neurol 2007; 66(8):732–739.

(335) Sarchielli P, Greco L, Floridi A et al. Excitatory amino acids and multiple sclerosis: evidence from cerebrospinal fluid. Arch Neurol 2003; 60(8):1082–1088.

(336) Sarchielli P, Greco L, Stipa A et al. Brain-derived neurotrophic factor in patients with multiple sclerosis. J Neuroimmunol 2002; 132(1–2):180–188.

(337) Vercellino M, Merola A, Piacentino C et al. Altered glutamate reuptake in relapsing-remitting and secondary progressive multiple sclerosis cortex: correlation with microglia infiltration, demyelination, and neuronal and synaptic damage. J Neuropathol Exp Neurol 2007; 66(8):732–739.

(338) Basso AS, Frenkel D, Quintana FJ et al. Reversal of axonal loss and disability in a mouse model of progressive multiple sclerosis. J Clin Invest 2008; 118(4):1532–1543.

(339) Sandyk R, Iacono RP. Improvement by picoTesla range magnetic fields of perceptual-motor performance and visual memory in a patient

with chronic progressive multiple sclerosis. Int J Neurosci 1994; 78(1–2):53–66.

(340) Sandyk R, Derpapas K. Magnetic fields normalize visual evoked potentials and brainstem auditory evoked potentials in multiple sclerosis. Int J Neurosci 1993; 68(3–4):241–253.

(341) Sandyk R. Rapid normalization of visual evoked potentials by picoTesla range magnetic fields in chronic progressive multiple sclerosis. Int J Neurosci 1994; 77(3–4):243–259.

(342) Sandyk R. Resolution of sleep paralysis by weak electromagnetic fields in a patient with multiple sclerosis. Int J Neurosci 1997; 90(3–4):145–157.

(343) Sandyk R. Reversal of visuospatial hemi-inattention in patients with chronic progressive multiple sclerosis by treatment with weak electromagnetic fields. Int J Neurosci 1994; 79(3–4):169–184.

(344) Sandyk R. Successful treatment of multiple sclerosis with magnetic fields. Int J Neurosci 1992; 66(3–4):237–250.

(345) Sandyk R. Treatment with electromagnetic field alters the clinical course of chronic progressive multiple sclerosis--a case report. Int J Neurosci 1996; 88(1–2):75–82.

(346) Sandyk R. Treatment with electromagnetic fields reverses the long-term clinical course of a patient with chronic progressive multiple sclerosis. Int J Neurosci 1997; 90(3–4):177–185.

(347) Sandyk R, Iacono RP. Improvement by picoTesla range magnetic fields of perceptual-motor performance and visual memory in a patient with chronic progressive multiple sclerosis. Int J Neurosci 1994; 78(1–2):53–66.

(348) Sandyk R, Derpapas K. Magnetic fields normalize visual evoked potentials and brainstem auditory evoked potentials in multiple sclerosis. Int J Neurosci 1993; 68(3–4):241–253.

(349) Sandyk R. Rapid normalization of visual evoked potentials by picoTesla range magnetic fields in chronic progressive multiple sclerosis. Int J Neurosci 1994; 77(3–4):243–259.

(350) Sandyk R. Resolution of sleep paralysis by weak electromagnetic fields in a patient with multiple sclerosis. Int J Neurosci 1997; 90(3–4):145–157.

(351) Sandyk R. Reversal of visuospatial hemi-inattention in patients with chronic progressive multiple sclerosis by treatment with weak electromagnetic fields. Int J Neurosci 1994; 79(3–4):169-184.

(352) Sandyk R. Successful treatment of multiple sclerosis with magnetic fields. Int J Neurosci 1992; 66(3–4):237-250.

(353) Sandyk R. Treatment with electromagnetic field alters the clinical course of chronic progressive multiple sclerosis--a case report. Int J Neurosci 1996; 88(1–2):75–82.

(354) Sandyk R. Treatment with electromagnetic fields reverses the long-term clinical course of a patient with chronic progressive multiple sclerosis. Int J Neurosci 1997; 90(3–4):177–185.

(355) Crevenna R, Mayr W, Keilani M et al. Safety of a combined strength and endurance training using neuromuscular electrical stimulation of thigh muscles in patients with heart failure and bipolar sensing cardiac pacemakers. Wien Klin Wochenschr 2003; 115(19–20):710-714.

(356) Quittan M, Wiesinger GF, Sturm B et al. Improvement of thigh muscles by neuromuscular electrical stimulation in patients with refractory heart failure: a single-blind, randomized, controlled trial. Am J Phys Med Rehabil 2001; 80(3):206–214.

(357) Quittan M, Sochor A, Wiesinger GF et al. Strength improvement of knee extensor muscles in patients with chronic heart failure by neuromuscular electrical stimulation. Artif Organs 1999; 23(5):432–435.

(358) Sillen MJ, Speksnijder CM, Eterman RM et al. Effects of neuromuscular electrical stimulation of muscles of ambulation in patients with chronic heart failure or COPD: a systematic review of the English-language literature. Chest 2009; 136(1):44–61.

(359) Crevenna R, Marosi C, Schmidinger M et al. Neuromuscular electrical stimulation for a patient with metastatic lung cancer--a case report. Support Care Cancer 2006; 14(9):970–973.

(360) Hascakova-Bartova R, Dinant JF, Parent A et al. Neuromuscular electrical stimulation of completely paralyzed abdominal muscles in spinal cord-injured patients: a pilot study. Spinal Cord 2008; 46(6):445–450.

(361) Maddocks M, Lewis M, Chauhan A et al. Randomized controlled pilot study of neuromuscular electrical stimulation of the quadriceps in patients with non-small cell lung cancer. J Pain Symptom Manage 2009; 38(6):950–956.

(362) Vrbova G, Hudlicka O, Centofanti KS. Application of Musce/Nerve Stimulation in Health and Disease. Birmingham, UK: Springer Science + Business Media B.V., 2008

Please Note

The suggested use of foods, supplements, and the discussion of electrical therapy and other interventions in this book are not meant to be medical advice and should not replace the receipt of medical care from a qualified personal physician. There is always the potential for interactions with your other issues and medicines that you are taking. It is very important to talk with your physician about any supplements, diet changes, or other interventions prior to starting them, to avoid adverse reactions, some of which could be very serious or even deadly.

Research Opportunity

Please help me conduct research on the impact of intensive nutrition and neuromuscular electrical stimulation in others. If you are going to attempt to emulate the interventions I used so successfully to restore my health, please go to my Web site, www.terrywahls.com, and participate in the longitudinal surveys. The more people that I have completing the surveys of the use of intensive nutrition and electrical stimulation over time, the sooner I will have publishable information on their use in the setting of multiple sclerosis. That is important, because it will be through reading peer-reviewed scientific publications that the medical community decides what treatments are appropriate for their patients. Therefore, each of you who reads this book can have an important role to play in determining how effective and safe the use of intensive, directed nutrition and neuromuscular electrical stimulation is.

Dr. Wahls MS News
Dr. Wahls MS News is an electronic newsletter in which Dr. Wahls reviews the role of specific nutrients, electrotherapy, and other news in the treatment of multiple sclerosis and neurodegenerative conditions. Many will find that improving their nutrition for brain health is good for their bodies, as well as their emotions. More information can found at www.terrywahls.com.

Other works by Terry L. Wahls, M.D.

The Primer Never Written
Audio CD

Dr. Wahls reads a number of essays about the interface between being a patient, a physician, and a family member.

Up from the Chair
Audio CD

Dr. Wahls reads essays about having multiple sclerosis and her descent into a progressively severe disability, and her remarkable ascent back to the walking world. These essays include reflections on the role nutrition plays in the burden of chronic disease in our children and in America.

Visit her Web site: **www.terrywahls.com**

About the Author

After four years in a wheelchair and an electric scooter, Dr. Wahls studied the medical literature. Eventually, she devised a new theory about progressive MS. She tested that theory on herself, with amazing results. After a year with this new treatment protocol based upon electricity and nutrition, she now routinely rides her bicycle eight miles at a time, including hills.

She is completing Up From the Chair, Defeating Secondary Progressive MS: a rich look into living with multiple sclerosis, coping with the progressive loss of self, and the interventions which restored her strength. News about her progress can be found on her Web site: www.terrywahls.com

Other educational materials are available through her Web site: **www. terrywahls.com**, including the Food as Medicine course.

Media Presentations

Dr. Wahls is available for workshops and lectures on Food as Medicine. Please contact Dr. Wahls through her Web site.

Order more copies of this book by contacting:

TZ Press, L.L.C.
Suite #101
1215 Santa Fe Drive
Iowa City, Iowa 52246-8638
U.S.A.

Index

Note: An 'n' after a page number indicates a footnote; 'f' indicates a figure; and 't' indicates a table.

Printed in Great Britain
by Amazon.co.uk, Ltd.,
Marston Gate.